THE
KTHROUGH
TEP PLAN

STOP DIETING. START LIVING.

FAT MADNESS

HOW TO STOP THE DIET CYCLE AND ACHIEVE PERMANENT WELL-BEING

PHILLIP M. SINAIKIN, M.D.
WITH JUDITH SACHS
AUTHORS OF *AFTER THE FAST*

FAT
MADNESS

FAT MADNESS

How to Stop the Diet Cycle and Achieve Permanent Well-being

PHILLIP M. SINAIKIN, M.D.

WITH JUDITH SACHS

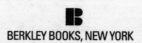

BERKLEY BOOKS, NEW YORK

FAT MADNESS

A Berkley Book / published by arrangement with
Phillip M. Sinaikin, M.D.

PRINTING HISTORY
Berkley trade paperback edition / March 1994

ISBN: 0-425-14103-9

BERKLEY®
Berkley Books are published by The Berkley Publishing Group,
200 Madison Avenue, New York, New York 10016.
BERKLEY and the "B" design
are trademarks belonging to the Berkley Publishing Corporation.

PRINTED IN THE UNITED STATES OF AMERICA

10 9 8 7 6 5 4 3 2 1

I lovingly dedicate this book to my wife, Ronnie, and my three daughters: Jamie, Benay, and Shara. I also dedicate this book to all of those who work in and benefit from caring about people in recovery.

—P.S.

For my *sensei*s—Deborah Jowitt, Alvin Ailey, Alan Levy, Dr. Stephen Gushin, and Susanna and Guy DeRosa—who have all helped to show me that you must start with the mind to get to the body.

—J.S.

Acknowledgments

I want to thank my always supportive literary agent and very good friend Susan Ginsburg for all of her help, faith, and encouragement, especially through the tough times. I also want to thank my editor Elizabeth Beier for her generosity and assistance. Finally I want to thank my writer and friend Judith Sachs for her inspirations, ideas, and marvelous writing.

—P.S.

Contents

The Nine-Step Fat Madness Recovery Program

STEP 1: *I admit that I don't know how to control my weight.*

STEP 2: *I must learn more about my body and food.*

STEP 3: *I accept the need to let go of myths and false hopes about my body.*

STEP 4: *I recognize that I must approach weight loss in a rational way.*

STEP 5: *I know that losing pounds is only the beginning.*

STEP 6: *I understand that lasting success requires true change.*

STEP 7: *I will no longer be a victim.*

STEP 8: *I will take care of myself for myself.*

STEP 9: *I fully accept the results of my best efforts.*

FAT
MADNESS

◼ INTRODUCTION

What Is Fat Madness?

How do you think about yourself? What's your opinion of your body? If you're like most people out there, you think you're overweight. Now wait a second—what's the key word in that last sentence? Is it *overweight*? No, it's *think*. You think, therefore, you are.

I don't care whether you're actually 50 or 100 pounds overweight, or whether you're below the standard weight table range for your height. I am willing to bet that your greatest obsession in life is controlling your weight. And I am also willing to wager that weight control, or your lack of it, is also your greatest source of failure and low self-esteem. The reason for this is that being overweight is not the number-one *physical* health problem in the United States, its the number-one *mental* health problem.

Can you stand back a minute and see the obsession with weight gripping those around you? You must have countless conversations with close friends and total strangers about the latest way to keep pounds off—and I'm sure one thing you all have in common is failure. Failure to lose or to maintain weight loss is a national preoccupation. But why? Do you know that you are living in a society that spends over 30 billion dollars a year on weight control and yet is getting fatter every year?

Then you know that it is time for something new, a radically different approach to the problem of body-weight obsession and weight-control failure. You are holding that radically different program in your hands right now.

1

If you have purchased this book in the hope that at last, here is a diet that will really do it for you—take the weight off and keep it off, make you trim and thin, and change your entire life— you've bought the wrong book.

You have not purchased a carrot-before-the-horse, promise-of-heaven-in-a-few-pounds diet book. This is not a book designed to help you mold and shape your body into the idealized perfect form you've been brainwashed to want. This is, rather, a book intended to tone and shape your *mind* so you won't be obsessed with weight control. It is, in fact, a mind-shaping book. When you learn to think clearly and rationally about your body and the food you put in it, and when you learn how to recapture your lost feelings of self-worth, successful long-term weight control will automatically follow.

Why do you think you need another new diet plan, anyway? For heaven's sake, you're already an expert on low-fat, high-carb, meal substitution, high-pro, low-pro diets. You know your calories and grams of fat by heart; you are an authority on how much you can cheat and not have it register on the scale.

You already know the heartbreak of falling off the diet, ignoring the weight gain for a while and then, when your clothes start to get tight and the sense of fullness and discomfort creeps up on you, how hopelessness settles in again.

You blew it. You lost. You failed. What good is it anyway, you say? That diet wasn't right for me. It didn't work with my body's metabolism. It didn't satisfy my cravings for certain tastes. It never filled me up. And anyway, this was a terrible time for me to start trying to lose weight. My job's a mess, I can't meet a man (or, in another scenario, my husband's so critical), my life's a mess, I can't cope with all the hundreds of daily chores I'm expected to perform.

And then, as the weight settles down on you like a burden you felt destined to carry all your life, you resign yourself to it. This is me. I'll never be any thinner; I'll never get any better; my life can't improve because how could anyone listen to me, hire me, respect me, love me when I look the way I do? That's it. The End. *Finis*.

Then you happen to be watching television or reading a magazine or wandering through a bookstore and a promise of youthful vitality and gorgeous slimness pops out at you. That model looks so fabulous, so radiant—so happy! You could be like her. You just didn't try hard enough last time. This time you'll *get it*. This time it's going to work for you.

So you pick up the latest diet book or product and give it a whirl. One more time you're on the weight-loss roller-coaster.

STOP! This is nuts! It's insanity. It is, in fact, Fat Madness.

Fat Madness is an intense, all-consuming preoccupation with body weight, size, shape, food, and dieting. It's based on a distorted perception of yourself, a vision perpetrated by society and history and the media. Television shows, movies, and the multi-billion-dollar diet industry image-makers have promised you a quick fix, if only you'd change your body. The propaganda we're all fed daily has succeeded in draining overweight people and people who just think they're overweight of their sense of self-worth and personal effectiveness.

This information doesn't just hit us when we're old enough to understand a print ad or a television commercial. It's fed to us from our earliest days by those who love us. Your own family conspired in this terrible disease of self-loathing, even if they didn't do it intentionally. The messages you got from parents ("Susie's the smart one; Carol's the skinny beauty.") and your peers ("My belly is okay but I can't even try on bathing suits because my thighs give me the creeps.") all sank in and became part of your belief system. You've been systematically programmed to believe that it's not just desirable but essential to stay slim and trim in order to attract the opposite sex, get ahead in life, and be ecstatic and euphoric by turning into some ideal that is ultimately impossible to achieve.

The corollary to this way of thinking is that the demon is food. If you eat it, you get fat and ugly; if you stop eating it, you get slim and devastating. Then, and only then, will you be happy. Women are particular victims of this lopsided kind of thinking, but in these days of steroid rage and sculpted muscles, even men have succumbed to the lure of Fat Madness.

In order to reach this illusive nirvana, you've dieted, then gained back when the slimmer weight didn't give you that euphoria you imagined it would provide, and tried another diet. And another. Frustrated and noncompliant, you failed again and again, only to try once more with renewed hope that *just this one final time* you'd be successful.

The notion that if you change your weight, you'll change your destiny, is a very appealing one. If, in fact, all you had to do was diet successfully and get thin to make your life change drastically, the world would be a different place.

Of course you know when you stop to think rationally and realistically that this is total bunk. The way you look doesn't guarantee that you will succeed in life, and it certainly doesn't directly determine whether you will be an upbeat, positive person or a desperate, negative one. Physically handicapped people can exude confidence and self-esteeem; yet some of the thinnest, most classically "beautiful" people can have the worst self-images and negative attitudes.

Everything feeds in (if you'll pardon the expression) to the encouragement of Fat Madness. There are those ads with anorexic models hawking diet products, and there are those television shows with people testifying to losing hundreds of pounds in just a few months. There are prepackaged food programs, conveniently offered so that you don't have to make any choices about what you put into your body. There are books by experts that will advise you to deny yourself favorite foods that are "bad" for you and only eat the bland uninteresting foods they say are "good." Soon, you come to define yourself as good or bad based solely on your compliance with these arbitrary rules of abstinence. Look at it logically for a second: "Good" and "bad" are heavily weighted moral pronouncements. Is eating a food that might put weight on you equivalent to committing a crime?

Thus dieting becomes the ultimate achievement, where your self-worth is equated with your ability to resist food and cope with deprivation. You can't even go out to a nice restaurant every once in a while and enjoy yourself. You have to watch out for the dangers lurking close by, ready to strike. Dangers like sauces, fried foods, marbled steaks, white flour, sugar, desserts, and dripping-in-butter delights.

The way to think about body image has been drilled into you over and over throughout your life. If you're less than perfect (unless you're Oprah or Roseanne, and even they have problems with their self-images), you're doomed, according to the popular message. If you're fat, if you feel fat, if something bulges or if something isn't tight and taut, you need help. You need a diet.

I'm here to tell you that there is another way out of this insanity. Let's face it, you need another diet like you need a hole in the head. What you really need is to rebuild your self-esteem, and there's only one way to do that. It has very little to do with what the scale or the mirror tells you about yourself. Rather, it has to do with turning inward, to the source of all this emotion and self-defeating thinking that goes on inside you. Fat Madness is a sickness that you caught early on and never recovered from. In a way, you didn't want to get better from thinking so badly about yourself, because it made such great sense. After all, no one ever tried to teach you to feel better, only to look better. And when it seems the whole world is in perfect agreement, how in God's name are you supposed to figure out for yourself that things could—or should—be different?

Now it's time to see the cyclical dieting you've done throughout your life as a symptom of a greater illness—that of not trusting yourself or liking yourself. Once you can recover from Fat Madness, you'll be on the path to a very positive and healthy life.

Recovery is a systematic, step-by-step deprogramming of the brainwashing you have undergone for longer than you can recall. The fact that you can't recall it is significant, because it shows how insidious and covert this process is. Recovery is a method of self-healing that not only helps you to make positive and permanent changes in your behaviors but to also make positive and permanent changes in your self-image and outlook on life.

Recovery is the process that helps alcoholics stop drinking for good, helps gamblers stop gambling for good, and helps people who are crippled by negative emotions feel better about themselves for good. With weight control, the problem isn't losing weight, its keeping the weight off for good. We can learn from the addicts and gamblers. I have. I have treated addiction for eight years. The Nine-Step Fat Madness Recovery Program is a system I designed specifically for chronic, unsuccessful dieters like yourself.

When I speak of *recovery,* I mean the long and slow process of wresting your mind, body, and emotions from the grips of a very potent disease syndrome. In order to get better, you will first be asked to acknowledge fully and honestly the true nature of your disease, Fat Madness (Step 1). You will then be educated about the biological and social forces that have brought you to where you are today (Step 2). Then I will ask you to begin to let go of false hopes and beliefs about your body and your weight (Step 3). This will prepare you to make sane and intelligent choices in Steps 4 and 5 where we will deal with practical ways to lose weight. This will bring us to the most important step (Step 6) where I will teach you simple yet highly effective techniques to maintain a weight loss for life.

You still have further to go in the recovery process. Weight maintenance is not the end of the road. Even the most sensible and reasonable long-term behavior changes can falter in the grip of lingering feelings of self-doubt and fear. In Steps 7, 8, and 9, we will work together to undo fully and irrevocably the damage Fat Madness has done to you. In these last vital steps you—and you alone—will immunize yourself from its insidious damage for good.

Recovery is not an easy process. Although the step program described in this book is not the same as the one used for recovery from alcohol and drug addiction, you will find certain similarities. Eating is not an addiction; it is an activity necessary to survival. However, the mechanisms of behavior that surround chronic dieting do bear certain resemblances to those used by alcoholics and drug abusers. Getting rid of the substance is not your goal. You want to get rid of the fear, pain, and anxiety that make you repeat the same old destructive behaviors again and again.

Understand that losing weight will not fulfill your own personal dream, allow you to win the Nobel prize or earn a million dollars or wind up in the happiest marriage this side of heaven. Once you have gained control over your Fat Madness, you will be moving toward something far richer, far more long-lasting: peace of mind.

It is this great, calming force—accessible to all of us—toward which I direct you now. Relax. Take your time. Heal yourself.

—PHILLIP M. SINAIKIN, M.D.
Longwood, Florida 1994

I Admit That I Don't Know How to Control My Weight

Janet is a twenty-year-old college junior who stands five feet six inches tall and weights 137 pounds. For as long as she can remember, she's been bottom-heavy, just like her mom. She carries most of her fat in her hips and thighs, giving her a sort of "water bottle" figure, which she loathes and despises. It is, to her way of thinking, the biggest obstacle in her life. And it affects everything she does, every decision she makes.

It's 7:00 A.M. Janet gets up for a day filled with biology and business classes, lunch with friends at the pizza shop, and a sorority rush party in the evening. But before the day begins, there is a ritual she must perform.

Janet gets out of bed and goes directly to the bathroom. She's thirsty, but she won't take a glass of water—not yet. She sits on the toilet, urinating with a purpose. She's done in only ten seconds, and then she glances into the bowl. The water is now dark yellow, almost orange. She sits down again, forcefully squeezing, but manages only a few more drops.

"Damn, where the hell is all that water I drank last night?" She tries desperately to move her bowels, but can't. "I'll allow a pound for that," she thinks. She wants her shower, but won't take it yet, can't get dry enough after a shower, her hair's really heavy, and she can't be sure some hidden, clinging water on other parts of her body won't add some extra weight. She strips off her pajamas, then her panties, and with trepidation, she steps up on the scale. "I hate this," she says to herself.

She stands up on her toes, the numbers whirl, but for a fraction of a second she catches sight of 130; then the pointer zooms up. For a moment, she considers jumping off the scale, not facing the hideous truth. After all, she swore she was only going to weigh herself every two weeks when she started her new diet three days ago. (She's stood on the scale eighteen times since then.) Yesterday she bummed a water pill from a friend and last night she was 135, which was 2 pounds less than in the morning, but thirst had gotten the best of her and she had two cans of Diet Coke before bed and two glasses of water during the night. "I'll pee it out in the morning," she predicted.

The scale comes to a stop at 137—well, really 136 ¾. Still on her toes, she shifts her weight from one foot to the other, then rocks back on her heels, finally finding a position where the scale inches down to 135 ½. "Okay, I've only gained half a pound." But then, in a wave of masochism, she plops both feet flat on the scale and watches it settle at 137 ½. She jumps off, curses, kicks the scale against the wall, adding another dent to the already mutilated little machine and a chip off the bathroom tile.

She gets into the shower now, letting the hot water course down her shoulders. It would feel great if she weren't so depressed. There's only one thing on Janet's mind: "I gotta get serious today. Maybe I'll fast, at least skip lunch, maybe another water pill, no breakfast for sure. God, I'm hungry!"

To reassure herself, she runs her hands over her tummy. She's worked so hard to get it flat, it's usually her pride and joy, but today it's bulging. A brief lapse in concentration, that's all. She sucks it back in, back into the shape in which it remains for all the world to see, a self-imposed girdle. The only place she ever lets it out is in gym where it's physically impossible to breathe hard and hold your stomach in at the same time.

She lifts her leg to wash her calf, but focuses instead on her thigh. That hideous thigh. A balloon filled with grape jelly would be firmer than that thigh. She can hardly stand to look at it, the mammoth bulges of unadulterated fat, the moon craters of cellulite. She pulls the skin on her thigh out with both hands, which smoothes the inner thigh into an unwrinkled line from knee to groin. "Sexy," she murmurs. "No man could resist that thigh." But then her wet, soapy hands lose their grip on the skin and her inner thigh is instantly transformed back into its fat, wrinkled, not-even-a-blind-man-would-touch-it natural shape.

Janet tries not to think about it anymore. She quickly finishes her shower, silently reviewing the biology chapter she studied last night. "I really like biology," she allows herself to think in that brief moment. Time for classes soon, time to get dressed. But there is one more irresistible ritual to perform before she faces the world.

She drops her towel and stands in front of the full-length mirror mounted on the closet door. The picture cut from *Cosmopolitan* stares mockingly from the top left corner. Totally nude, Janet takes stock of herself, doing a running inventory of every nook and cranny. Breasts, okay: They stand up straight and firm, unmarred by stretch marks or puckers. She lifts her left arm and with her right hand strikes the skin hanging from the tricep. It wiggles like Jell-O. She angrily drops her arm, casts a quick glance at her firm, sucked-in belly, then lowers her gaze to the "horror." From her thin waist, her hips swell like two saddlebags of flesh. Her thighs meet at her groin and her legs don't part company until her ankles. Thunder thighs.

She turns sideways. Her bottom looks like two basketballs pressed together. She smacks a cheek—Jell-O again! "Enough meat there to feed the whole college." Then, in a final gesture of self-mockery, she puffs her cheeks, sticks out her belly, and with tears welling in her eyes, screams, *"You fat pig!"*

Totally demoralized now, her mind racing with thoughts of food and fat, her stomach churning with hunger, she turns from the mirror to the totally depressing task of dressing. No designer jeans for her, no clinging shorts or Lycra bodysuits. Her drawer is filled with loose-fitting, fat-hiding, non–curve-defining sweats. She struggles into the pants, tying the drawstring loosely, then quickly covers up with the shapeless top, size XL so it will come down over her hips and thighs. She yanks on a pair of Adidas and ties the laces, doesn't bother with her hair. Forget makeup, what's the use? On the way out of the room, she glances at her biology project on the desk, the one with the A+ on it, the one on top of her latest dean's letter, commending her for her excellent grades. "Big frigging deal!" she growls, slamming the door behind her. "Will I ever be 115?"

Feelings About the Body Cancel Out Rational Thought and Behavior

Janet has repeated these awful morning exercises, with very little variation, every day for the past three years. If you looked at her, you would see none of the "horror" that is so clearly evident to her. She would seem, instead, a normal-sized young woman with a non-hourglass figure, rounder and wider below her waist than above. But for Janet, her body's shape and size is a cruel trick on the part of Mother Nature. She is tormented by one terrible thought: No matter how hard she tries, she will never weigh the right amount.

But what is "the right amount"? It should be pretty clear that 115 wouldn't do it for her. Nor would 110. Nor would any weight known to man. Even if she were emaciated, her hips and thighs would still appear large in comparison to the rest of her body, and she would be dissatisfied with the shape of her body.

Janet is in the throes of Fat Madness. In order to escape from its clutches, she is going to have to take steps to change her mind. In the course of following the program, her body will change as well, but that will not be the only measure of success that she's aiming for by the time she reaches Step 9. If she fully understands and uses the program I will outline in this book, her weight and shape will no longer be of primary importance in her life.

Janet's real problem has nothing to do with her weight or her shape. She is chronically miserable with the way she turned out, and because she doesn't feel okay in her body, nothing else in her life can turn out well for her. She can't be smart, sexy, popular, or successful—according to her—because she looks the way she does and can't alter it.

What she has to do first is admit to herself that her *feelings* about her physical form have for a very long time stood in the way of *acting* in a rational manner about establishing good weight control habits. The next thing she has to do is acknowledge that she is her own worst enemy in controlling her weight because she believes that she is doomed to fail. When you're sure you can't do something, amazingly enough, you can't.

Denial: The Easy Way Out

Denial is a central concept in the treatment of addiction. You've probably heard of the alcoholic or drug addict being "in denial." This refers to the fact that they refuse to admit that they have a problem with alcohol or drugs even when their problem is painfully obvious to everyone around them. Overcoming this denial is the first step in recovery from alcoholism or drug addiction.

You now need to understand that denial is also alive and well in the chronic dieter. That denial is characterized by blaming everything and everyone but yourself for your problem with weight. The hard truth you must now acknowledge is that *it's not the diet, it's the dieter*.

Denial in the chronic dieter has its roots in a sense of powerlessness over the self-hating side of yourself. You probably aren't aware that it's there, but it pervades everything you do and are. It doesn't make a difference whether you're forty pounds overweight or five, whether you are slightly underweight for your build or whether you simply hate part of your body. If you deny that your self-defeating attitude is what makes you fail each time you try to diet, you can never proceed beyond the dismal realization that you will never achieve what you want to in life.

See how denial is a vicious cycle? If you feel that all of life's bounties will only come to you when you weigh a certain number of pounds or feel that others expect you to look a certain way, and yet you are never happy with the results of any diet you've ever been on, then how can you reach your dream? Like Janet, you go down a few pounds, then rebound a few, and are immediately convinced that you're going backward—that you will never stop regressing. So you give up on the diet (no matter which plan you're on) and you gain back more than you lost the last time you starved yourself.

It is your unwillingness to comply with sensible eating and exercising, not the program itself, that keeps your scale reading the same or higher each day. As long as you keep insisting that it's the diet plan or the time of month or the particular man you're involved with or the miserable job you're in that keeps you from taking off weight and keeping it off, you're in denial.

It doesn't matter whether you've lost dozens of pounds and failed to keep them off or the same five over and over again. You are repeating that old, well-known, unworkable mantra: If I could just lose _____ I'd be perfect. And it will never work for you.

Who Is the Real Enemy?

I want to tell you right now that you have within yourself all the resources you will ever need to win your own personal war. As soon as you recognize the enemy, you'll be in great shape.

The enemy is your self-loathing. It is not your flabby thighs or jelly underarms, not your weight or your figure. People who suffer from Fat Madness don't always have an unmanageable problem with eating, but instead, have a chronic problem with compliance and long-term positive behavior change. Understand that you aren't an addict abusing a dangerous drug. An addict is someone hooked on a substance that is disease-promoting, such as alcohol or drugs. You can live without booze or grass, but you can't live without food. And food is certainly not a dangerous or addictive substance. It only seems life-threatening in your way of thinking because it offers a convenient excuse for what's holding up everything else in your life.

Once you start seeing the enemy as your unwillingness to make vital lifestyle changes, you're on the road to recovery. It's that important moment when you stop denying that you have a problem that the problem starts to take a shape you can hold onto and work with.

The Two Levels of Denial

Denial is a complex issue and it is difficult to understand because it may occur on several levels at the same time.

You really know—every chronic dieter does—what is needed to lose weight and keep it off. If you believe that you could lose weight if only you could find someone, some book, some program, some divine inspiration that would make it all clear, then you are in denial. You are giving yourself the runaround.

Be real. You know all there is to know and more about the process of caloric intake and expenditure. You know about plateaus, about water weight, about diet burnout. You also know all about the importance of regular exercise and have probably started and stopped more exercise programs than you care to count.

However, the true reason you can't change is that you *think* you know why you don't stick to a weight maintenance program, but, in fact, you don't know. You think it is because you are powerless over tempting food or because you can't stand the tough demands of an exercise program, but you're wrong. These are emphatically not the reasons you fail. You aren't powerless over the lure of food or the rigors of exercise at all.

Chronic dieters are really powerless over their own self-defeating attitudes, beliefs, and feelings about their bodies and their self-worth. This type of denial is so insidious and so overwhelming that you can't be expected to grasp its many facets without taking a new perspective. In this nine-step program, you'll find doors opening into a different way of looking at your dieting and relapse patterns.

Think about the word *powerless* for a minute. If you lack power, you're weak, ineffective, easily swayed. You can be bowled over by anything and anyone, including the next diet guru as well as the next ad for the best-tasting, most luscious chocolate mousse ever to appear in your supermarket's freezer case.

A belief in your own powerlessness robs you of your birthright and your natural ability to act on your own. Of course you hate to acknowledge that there's a part of yourself that you can't change: You'd rather have someone else do it for you. But if you are under the sway of Fat Madness, no one will do it for you the right way, so you're really stuck. If you can't do it, and no one else seems to have the answer for you, you will go right back to believing the message that society has been feeding you for a long, long time: You are right to feel terrible about your body and yourself.

Turn It Over

All right, maybe you can't do it alone. Maybe you are helpless in the face of these awful feelings and you do need help. The first step in recovery is to say, "Yes, I admit that I don't know what I'm doing here and I keep doing the same useless things over and over again. So now I'm going to turn my problem over to someone who can teach me why I can't come to grips with my weight problem and take care of it once and for all."

This is hard to think about because realizing that you can't do it yourself is frightening.

Take heart, because you can do it alone as soon as you understand your inner mechanisms and triggers. Your powerlessness can and will be conquered by a fearless exploration of yourself, on which you are about to embark. Along the way you will gain greater understanding of the irrational and self-defeating person you've become in your illusive search to look and be a certain way.

The Diet Industry

You haven't fallen into Fat Madness all by yourself; you've been systematically molded and brainwashed into believing our culture's dictum: You can never be too thin or too rich.

Look at the pie graph below. (Given the way you think, pie graphs were invented by cruel statisticians who just wanted to remind you every time you looked at some data that you shouldn't be thinking about pie.)

See how many billions of dollars are netted each year trying to help people take off weight and stay thin. By the year 2000, the projection is that 55 billion dollars will be spent annually on the pursuit of perfect bodies. Between hospital-sponsored

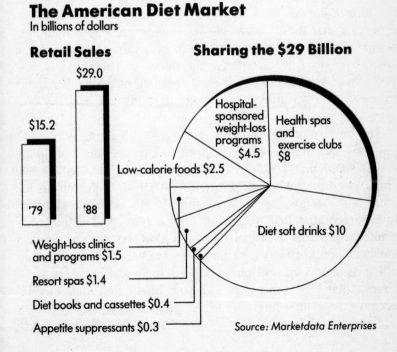

The American Diet Market
In billions of dollars

Retail Sales

$29.0

$15.2

'79   '88

Sharing the $29 Billion

Hospital-sponsored weight-loss programs $4.5

Health spas and exercise clubs $8

Low-calorie foods $2.5

Diet soft drinks $10

Weight-loss clinics and programs $1.5

Resort spas $1.4

Diet books and cassettes $0.4

Appetite suppressants $0.3

Source: Marketdata Enterprises

weight loss programs, private programs including those available on computer disk, diet products, frozen foods, appetite suppressants, long- and short-term stays at exclusive spas, books, and cassettes, many people are making many dollars on your obsession.

Even so, Americans are getting fatter each year: 45 million are charted as being overweight in 1993. That's 21 percent of the total population of the country! And 95 percent of all dieters gain back every pound they lose within five years of being on a program.

It's like beating your head against a wall, isn't it? Only in this industry, they don't let you feel so good when you stop. Everywhere you go, you receive messages—verbal and nonverbal, blatant and implied—of what you *should* look like, how healthy you *should* become, how sculpted your muscles *should* be. You've undoubtedly been told that thin people live longer, tolerate surgery and anesthesia better, and are able to concentrate for longer periods of time. I've even read come-ons for diet programs that make incredible statements such as that thinner people get into fewer accidents! You hear this stuff once and it sounds bogus. But if you're in the throes of Fat Madness, and you hear it over and over, it begins to sound plausible. You have to chew it over a little. Maybe you might just try that new program or product.

The only catch is, you try it, and you can't do it. Why don't you look like that model in the print ad after months of drinking a diet supplement? One reason may be that Madison Avenue employs women who fall in the lowest 10 to 15 percent of the ideal body weight curve. Many models are actually below the lowest recommended weight for their height. And if that emaciated image still isn't just right, the Madison Avenue product hawkers won't think twice about using twelve- and thirteen-year-old girls made up and photographed to look like women. Of course their hips don't look like your hips (even after dieting) because these little girls don't have adult hips yet!

Speaking of hips, if you examine those ads closely, you'll

notice that none of the models are facing full front to the camera. Their curves are posed at their most flattering angle. Try it some-time. Have someone take a shot of you in shorts or a bathing suit as you stand askew to the camera, one leg coyly thrust in front of the other. It will be the picture you most treasure—until you get out of the depths of Fat Madness—because your hips look so amazingly skinny, you can scarcely believe they belong to you.

They do. But so do those same hips, facing outward, that you will call fat until you reach the second half of the Fat Madness program. You see that you have been brainwashed and barraged by an industry bent on changing your mind about your body. But the focus is wrong, and deep down, you know it.

The problem is not with the diet, it is with the dieter. Under-stand, please, that I'm not implying you are unmotivated or weak-willed. On the contrary, you have over the years exercised tremendous willpower, and have subjected yourself to one of worst experiences known to man—starvation. You have done this to yourself not once, but countless times because the diet industry says you should, and you believed them.

But what they have sold you, instead of the perfect diet that will allow you to control your weight permanently, is the carrot on the end of the stick that you can never reach. The product they sell is loss of pounds; but what you need is a way to change your habitual patterns of behavior. And this isn't a miracle food or a pill or a product you can hold in your hand. It is not a concrete, simple element but a whole new way of thinking about yourself and the world you live in.

The diet, fashion, entertainment, and advertising industries have given you messages that locked onto your brain with a death grip. The beliefs they have fed you have severely affected your ability to control your weight. Instead of helping, they have severely damaged you by selling you the wrong goods. Now you're going to get out of the clutches of this wrong thinking and turn yourself around so that instead of searching for the gold at the end of the rainbow, you will stumble on the rainbow itself.

How Do I Know I Have a Problem With Dieting?

Ask yourself, "Why can't I face a day with a total sense of well-being?"

Because you are deeply unsettled by your own sense of what you haven't accomplished as a dieter.

Because, no matter what the scale tells you, you don't believe it's helping.

Because no matter what you eat or don't eat, you hate your hips, your thighs, your stomach, your breasts—you fill in the blank.

The foundation of successful recovery of addicts is acknowledging that they are powerless in the face of their problem. Let's start there and move on.

Remember, your goal in this program is to find peace of mind and to like yourself—even love yourself. Before you can find peace, you must end the war you've been waging with food, with your body, with your mirror, and with your clothes.

Once you've admitted that all of the above sounds very familiar, you can admit that yes, you do have a Fat Madness obsession and you want to take care of it.

After that, change is possible.

Abilities: How Change Can Happen

Let's go back and look at Janet's story once again. In this scenario, Janet will have made the first inroads into her problem of denial.

She gets up and goes into the bathroom. First she urinates, then, because she's so thirsty, she has a glass of water.

What's different? Janet is taking care of her physical needs and isn't agonizing over body fantasies.

She takes off her pajamas and gets into the shower, thinking about the day ahead. She's curious about her weight but realizes that she's only been on her new diet for three days, so she probably has only lost water weight—if anything—by now and it would be depressing to see the numbers. She's going to wait until a week has passed to see how she's doing.

What's different? The weighing ritual is gone. Janet has a realistic appraisal of how diets work and knows herself well enough not to get back into demoralizing behavior around weight loss.

She feels incredibly hungry and decides to have a good, nourishing, high-fiber, low-fat breakfast. Because she's watching her weight, she decides that when she meets her friends at the pizza parlor for lunch, she'll have a big salad from the salad bar and one slice of pizza.

What's different? Janet is, once again, aware of her own needs and limitations. Since she's hungry now, she'll eat—but sensibly. And since she's complying with her diet, she's already planning what to have so that she can stick to her program. She won't force herself to eat bland, dull diet fare when her friends are having pizza. Instead, she'll enjoy the taste of something she really likes, but she'll limit her intake of it because it's highly caloric and ingesting more calories than she can burn off would be counter to her weight-loss goals.

Janet washes her body, enjoying the sensation of the washcloth on her skin. She admires her breasts (her best asset, she thinks—and others have agreed with her) and her stomach. It's been flatter when she's been at lower weights, but it's still a perfectly good part of her anatomy. She runs the washcloth over her hips and thighs, then her buttocks. Well, she wishes they were smaller and shapelier, but this is just a fact of life. Her bottom half is built like her mother's and nothing she can do will change that. She's gotten to the point where her hips and thighs don't repel her or attract her interest, particularly. They're just part of the whole.

She also knows that she's had problems staying with a diet in the past, and for that reason, she's larger all over than she'd like to be. But she knows that persistent good eating and exercising is going to take care of the excess poundage. And now, she's committed to that.

What's different? Janet is not obsessing about her individual good and bad parts, but enjoying the shower experience, enjoying the feeling of being naked and wet and at home in her body. She admits that she doesn't have a perfect body and never will, but she's reasonably satisfied with what she's got. She also admits her problem with dieting in the past and seems to be approaching it now from a different, more positive angle.

She towels off and walks into the bedroom, facing the mirror on the closet door. "Hi!" she says to her image. "What are you going to wear today?" She scans her selection of clothes, finally choosing a pair of jeans and a tailored shirt in a brilliant blue shade that complements her eyes. She highlights the look with a thin black belt that has a silver buckle. Then she brushes her thick brunette hair, catching it on the side with a silver clip. She applies some mascara and a little lipstick, and she's ready to face the world.

What's different? Janet enjoys adorning her body. Clothing is more than functional for her, and it's there, not to hide anything but to accentuate her form. She does the most with what she has.

The First Step Is the Hardest

We take many steps in our lives, some small, some monumental. They're like New Years' resolutions—absolutely unshakable when we first decide to tackle them, then, with time and all the pressures we face daily, a real challenge to be fought with and overcome. Finally, these resolutions either become part of our lives, hardly a step at all but simply a piece of the strong fabric, or they are discarded totally, relegated to the trash heap of outdated ideas we once tried on for size.

The first step, of all the steps we take in a process, is always the hardest. We've never done it before, so we face the unknown, terrified of failure. We have no real models to fall back on as guides and protectors, so we're unsure and confused as to how to proceed.

And how do we know, before we've taken that first step, that the others will follow logically? How can we really count on that step being the one that will make the difference?

We can't.

It doesn't mean we shouldn't try. Sometimes the best thing to do is look over the edge, take a deep breath, take the risk, sail out into space, and pray a lot.

The first step in the Fat Madness program is to acknowledge that you have a problem with dieting. You've gained and lost weight over and over throughout your life and deep down inside you know that this battle you've fought with your body can't be won, because you will never be as thin, as lovely, or as desirable as society has convinced you that you must be.

Finding Growth-Promoting Acts

Your negative, self-defeating attitude is about to melt away like a chocolate bar in the sun. You are going to proceed inexorably toward growth—growth as a person as well as a dieter. It's time to work on *you,* not on a diet program or promise. It's time to explore new vistas that will be challenging and breathtaking and useful in whichever part of your life you choose to use them.

The goal of the work in this book is to educate yourself about weight control, body image, and societal expectations, and to make educated and rational choices about what you choose to do about your body and your food choices for the rest of your life.

This is empowering. Self-effectiveness is a wonderful concept. As you work your way through the next eight steps of this program, you will see how each success sets up the field for another success, and another. If you do fall backward, you'll have the strength to get up and move on again. Instead of letting people and attitudes do things to you, you will be acting for yourself on yourself.

In AA's twelve-step program, the first maxim everyone learns is Easy Does It: When I can't accomplish all that I want to, I will slow my pace. I will stop and think. I will try not to grasp things all at once.

It took a long time to become truly infected with Fat Madness. Give yourself time to work your way out of it. Honest, it will come.

◩ STEP 2: KNOWLEDGE

I Must Learn More About My Body and Food

You know, of course, that ignorance isn't bliss. Ignorance is just putting on blinders and hoping for the best. It keeps you in the dark and dooms you to repeat the mistakes of the past.

But *knowledge* truly brings power. It gives you the tools you need to develop control over your situation and to say good-bye to Fat Madness forever.

So your next step in the Nine-Step Fat Madness Recovery Program is to acquire objective knowledge about your body and food. Some of what you learn in this chapter might be familiar, but many other facts will be startlingly new.

Objective knowledge (getting the straight facts) is a necessary component of recovery, but it's by no means sufficient to do the job. (If objective knowledge alone were all it took to beat an addictive behavior, then the ads on television and the plethora of articles and lectures about substance abuse would have wiped out drug addiction a long time ago.)

But objective information is essential to give you a good start on the road to recovery. It really empowers you. You can tell yourself off when you're wrong, because you know better. You can sit back, use your mind, and give yourself an informed health lecture whenever you're feeling that your emotions are out of control and your consumption of food hangs in the balance.

MIND VS. BODY: THE GREAT FOOD CONFUSION

Let's think about it this way. Anne is a chronic dieter. She reads popular magazines all the time, and the hodgepodge of diet "facts" she's got stored in her brain would fill a refrigerator. Anne is feeling edgy because she's so hungry all the time. She had just rapidly lost five pounds on a new fat-burning scheme. What she doesn't know is that four and a half of those pounds she lost in three days were just water.

Anne's husband is away on a business trip; her kids are at sleep-away camp for a month, and she and her much-too-thin-without-even-trying friend have just seen a movie. She was ravenous when she got to the theater since she'd purposely skipped dinner. After a brief mental debate at the movie snack counter, she opted for the medium-size popcorn, justifying it to herself because she ordered it without butter. After all, Anne knows for sure that popcorn is a good diet food. It made her pretty thirsty, so she had a large diet soda with it.

Now the film is over and it's nearly ten o'clock. Anne and her friend are being seated in a local Mexican restaurant where they decided to go for a quick bite.

Anne's mind: *I'm ravenous. I don't know why I'm so hungry. What I really want is a frozen margarita and nachos deluxe. But I know how disastrously caloric that would be. So I'll just have a light beer and chips with some guacamole. That should be OK.*

Anne's body: *I could use about 500 more calories for my daily 1,800-calorie requirement. A big salad would be nice, with a lot of water or a refreshing fruit drink to dilute all of that salt I got from the popcorn. And to ensure the appropriate balance of nutrients I need, a bean and rice combination for dinner would be perfect.*

See what's going on here? There's a war between Anne's

mind and her body for correct information, balance, and fulfilled desires. Anne's light beer and guacamole with chips won't be significantly less caloric than the margarita and nachos. (Besides, as we will learn later in this chapter, it's not simply the number of calories you're eating, it's the source of those calories and how your body uses them that makes a difference in fat storage.)

Because Anne won't have enough food to fill her up, she'll leave the restaurant (having watched her friend eat voraciously) dissatisfied and frustrated. And if she dares to weigh herself the next morning, she may find to her dismay that the salty popcorn and nacho chips made her so thirsty that she drank back the four and a half pounds of water she "lost" on her diet.

Obviously, Anne's hodgepodge of diet facts only confused the issue in this situation. Let's look at some of the mistakes she made.

Mistake #1. Anne chose a new fad diet from a women's magazine promising rapid weight loss. Despite years of dieting and first-hand knowledge that weight lost quickly is usually gained back quickly, she still bought into the magical myth that five pounds of fat can simply disappear in three days, never to return.

Mistake #2. Trying to accelerate the weight loss even further, Anne ate nothing before the movie, even though she knew (again, from years of dieting experience) that skipping a meal usually causes a late-night binge.

Mistake #3. Anne was sure her popcorn was "safe" to eat. She didn't know that movie-theater popcorn is full of fat and salt, even without added butter. She also didn't know that guacamole, made from avocados, is a high-fat food.

Mistake #4. She didn't listen to her body when it told her in no uncertain terms to eat something healthy and filling at the Mexican restaurant.

Mistake #5. Anne allowed herself to suffer unnecessary and excessive pain, self-hate, and hopelessness about her weight problem the following day when the scale informed her that almost all of her five pounds had returned.

Anne is a typical chronic dieter with Fat Madness. She ignores or forgets all the lessons she's learned from past diets. She also lacks some fundamental information about what kinds of food will help her to maintain her weight and the way in which her body processes all foods. She separates the concept of the food that goes into her mouth from the calories and fat that end up in her system. No wonder she falls prey to one diet scheme after the next!

Correcting the Dieting Errors of the Past

You and Anne are about to learn all you need to know about the biology of weight control. Combining this with all of the practical weight control experience you've had in the past will give you the firm knowledge base you will need to begin your recovery from Fat Madness.

THE BIOLOGICAL FACTS
ABOUT BODY WEIGHT REGULATION

Fat People Do Not Eat More Than Thin People

It is a well-documented fact that the number of calories ingested by obese people is not a whole lot greater than that of thin people. Some people may overeat for a period of time and put on weight, but they maintain that higher weight with the same intake as their skinny friends. So all people with weight problems are not gluttons who continually stuff themselves with food. Nor are all thin people smart and healthy eaters. In fact, whether you're thin or fat is no great predictor of whether you have good or bad eating habits. What *is* predictive of a particular eating pattern is whether you are a dieter or a nondieter.

Chronic dieters tend to develop eating patterns that can have a profoundly negative impact on weight control. Years of either being on or off a diet distorts the dieter's relationship with food and turns him or her into what researchers call a restrained eater. This means that any time the dieter eats anything at all, whether she's mildly hungry, not hungry at all, or ravenous, she mentally puts on the brakes in a chronic effort to lose weight. Also, restrained eaters typically rule out all favorite fattening foods when they are being "good." This wouldn't be a bad way to shed pounds and keep them off, of course, if the dieter could keep her mental brakes on forever, but most people can't.

The downside to restrained eating is breaking restraint. When a chronic dieter breaks restraint, all hell breaks loose. Those stored-up months of deprivation and loss unleash a mindless weight-gaining binge on all of the foods the dieter denied herself when she was being "good." Now she overconsumes fat-filled, sugar-laden items for days, weeks, even months, often until she has regained all of the weight that she lost on her most recent diet.

This pattern is sadly familiar to me from my work with patients I treat for substance abuse. It is exactly the same addictive pattern I've seen in gamblers, alcoholics, and drug addicts when they relapse. Their relapse behaviors are more destructive than any dieter's, of course, but you need to understand the nature of this pattern in order to grasp how really insidious Fat Madness is, and how it can be controlled.

Mentally restraining or forbidding an addictive behavior may work for you in the short run, but it is never a successful long-term solution and ultimately leads to relapse. So every time your diet counselor, book, or program suggested that all you'd have to do to maintain your new weight was "never eat another potato chip" or "throw away your ice-cream scoop," they were setting you up for failure.

In the Fat Madness recovery program, on the other hand, you are going to succeed. In Step 6, I'll introduce a new concept about what and how to eat so that you can truly enjoy food (even foods you've been told are completely and irrevocably forbidden) and still maintain a sensible weight loss. For now, let's get back to the facts and look at the food issue in more detail.

What Is Food All About?

What you put into your body will affect the way your body looks and the way you feel. Some factors that determine how much of what you put in gets used and how much gets stored as fat are:

Genetics. Certain people have faster metabolisms, certain people process nutrients differently, and certain people store fat more efficiently.

Exercise. The more you move, the more you can eat and not gain weight. Exercise delivers the oxygen to the body that it needs to burn fat.

Attitude. If you're constantly worried about food, you tend to develop unhealthy eating patterns such as binging at night, which will affect the way your body stores fat, among other factors.

Balance of nutrients. You need a little of everything. Honest.

In the context of Fat Madness rehabilitation, you have to know the facts about food and how it affects you. Basically, it's very simple. Eat a little bit of everything. Don't listen to new diet pundits telling you that this or that is "good" or "bad" for you. In Step 6, I'll outline exactly how to do this.

FACTS ABOUT CARBOHYDRATES

Everyone's diet is made up of three basic nutrients: carbohydrates, fats, and protein. Carbohydrates come in two varieties: *simple carbohydrates* (sugars) and *complex carbohydrates* (fruits, grains, and vegetables). *Fats* come in three types: saturated, unsaturated, and monounsaturated. Finally, *protein* comes from two sources, animal and vegetable. It's really crucial for you to understand the way that these three nutrients are processed by the body so that you can have the knowledge you need when you are thinking about why and how you need to change what you eat. What follows is a basic lesson in nutrition.

Here's a simple fact: food is fuel. The body is a complex biological machine and, like all machines, it needs fuel to run. Unlike most machines, the body would not physically survive without its fuel. It also needs raw materials to repair and restructure damaged or used elements in the body. So as well as being fuel, food also provides the wood and nails, as it were, for this construction job the body does on a consistent basis. A body without proper nutrients can't build new bone tissue or blood cells. It can't help heal a cut or start a baby off on the right foot. A body can't continue life without its requisite nutrients.

Simple vs. Complex Carbohydrates

Let's start by looking at *carbohydrates*. The basic building blocks of carbohydrates are the simple molecules *glucose* and *fructose*. All carbohydrates are made up of various combinations and numbers of fructose and/or glucose molecules. Simple carbohydrates (white table sugar, for example) are short chains of these molecules. Complex carbohydrates (spaghetti or wheat bread) are long chains of fructose and glucose, bound together.

The body doesn't know or care which type of carbohydrate you're eating because it can *only* use simple glucose or fructose molecules for fuel. Complex carbohydrates must always be broken down into simple carbohydrate molecules before they're used for fuel.

The body's primary fuels are these glucose and fructose molecules. After you've ingested a carbohydrate, it's broken down into simple molecules during the digestion process and is then delivered from the intestines to the bloodstream. At this point, the molecules can either be used immediately to serve the body's current energy needs or stored for future use.

Now here comes the important stuff: Carbohydrates can be stored in two different forms. A very limited amount can be stored in the muscles or liver as glycogen, a polysaccaride made from sugar, used for generating energy as heat. *The rest is converted to fat*. That's right, carbohydrates can be turned into fat. Fortunately, this does not happen so easily. About 25 percent of the energy contained in carbohydrates is used for the chemical processes required to turn carbohydrates into fat. Put another way, if you have an excess of 100 calories' worth of carbohydrates to be stored, only 75 will ultimately end up as fat since 25 calories will be burnt up in the conversion process.

How is this related to body weight? Fat is calorically dense. Every nine calories of fat weighs one gram (as opposed to the more efficient, more slender four and a half calories per gram of carbohydrate or protein). So every time nine calories of fat are stored, one gram is added to your body weight.

Why are complex carbohydrates good for you and simple carbohydrates merely fattening? Since the body breaks down all carbohydrates into glucose or fructose molecules before they enter the bloodstream, what difference does it make which form we eat them in? To understand this, you have to have some basic knowledge about *blood glucose levels*.

Blood Glucose Levels

At some point in your dieting career, your doctor probably checked your blood glucose level to find out how much glucose, or fuel, was in your bloodstream. This is a very important test to determine if you have diabetes, a condition in which your blood glucose level is too high. The body works best when there is a steady, moderate level of glucose in the blood, with no real rises or dips in the level. The sensation of hunger is related in large part to the rate of dropping blood glucose levels. If you have a steady level in your blood, your hunger never gets out of control. Some people who experience rapid drops in blood glucose levels develop a condition known as reactive hypoglycemia. They have to consume certain foods at well-spaced intervals so that they don't become anxious and physically weak, two typical symptoms of the disease.

Let's combine our new blood glucose knowledge with our carbohydrate breakdown information. It's sort of a tortoise and hare story.

Simple carbohydrates, like rabbits, race to the finish line. When you eat a candy bar, the short chain of molecules doesn't take much time at all to break down, so glucose is rapidly absorbed into the bloodstream, giving you a sudden and walloping rise in blood glucose.

Because everything that goes up must come down, the peak is followed by a sharp dip, and you get hungry all over again. That candy bar you ate an hour ago is a fleeting memory on your tongue and you crave another one (or a doughnut, if no candy is available).

Long chains of glucose and fructose (complex carbohydrates) are the slow and steady tortoises. They take their own good time being broken down into their constituent glucose or fructose molecules because there are more of them, so they enter the bloodstream slowly and evenly. The steady stream of fuel delivered to the blood by a nice snack of hearty, seven-grain bread (no butter) without any peaks and valleys means you won't be hungry for another three hours or so.

Finally, complex carbohydrates come in foods that usually contain other important nutrients such as fiber, protein, and vitamins. Here is a chart summarizing the carbohydrate story:

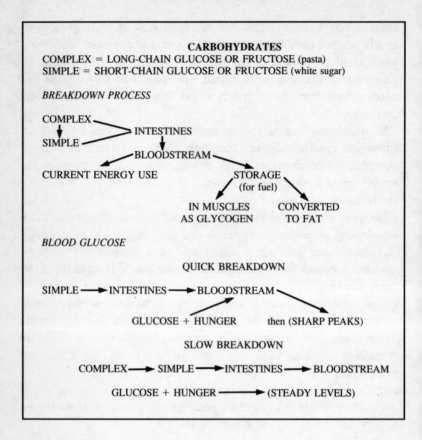

CARBOHYDRATES
COMPLEX = LONG-CHAIN GLUCOSE OR FRUCTOSE (pasta)
SIMPLE = SHORT-CHAIN GLUCOSE OR FRUCTOSE (white sugar)

BREAKDOWN PROCESS

COMPLEX
    ↓   INTESTINES
SIMPLE
                        ↓
                    BLOODSTREAM
CURRENT ENERGY USE   STORAGE
                                      (for fuel)
                            IN MUSCLES   CONVERTED
                            AS GLYCOGEN   TO FAT

BLOOD GLUCOSE

                    QUICK BREAKDOWN

SIMPLE ——→ INTESTINES ——→ BLOODSTREAM
                        GLUCOSE + HUNGER   then (SHARP PEAKS)

                    SLOW BREAKDOWN

COMPLEX ——→ SIMPLE ——→ INTESTINES ——→ BLOODSTREAM
GLUCOSE + HUNGER ————→ (STEADY LEVELS)

FACTS ABOUT FAT

Fat is a necessary nutrient for survival: *You cannot stay alive without consuming fat.* Fat cushions and insulates the tissues and internal organs of your body. Without a reasonable amount of fat, a woman's menstrual cycle and reproductive capacity is thrown completely out of whack. So regardless of fashion, regardless of all the anorexic models you see portrayed in ads and the barrage of anti-fat propaganda around you, you must take a reasonable stand when it comes to fat. Of course it shouldn't be abused, but it must be used properly.

Although it is essential to consume some fat in order to survive, you can live with a lot less fat than most people usually eat. The digestion of fat is a very complex process, and you don't really need all the details to grasp the essentials. So I'll skip to the chase and explain how digested fat is used by the body.

I mentioned earlier that food is both a fuel and a source of raw materials for the body. Fat's most essential role is as a raw material: Fats are a very important structural material in the membranes of every one of your billions of cells. Fats are also involved in the absorption of some very important vitamins, and they serve as the precursors or front-runners, if you will, for the hormones and other enzymes your body uses.

Fat is also a fuel that can be stored in an extremely efficient manner because it contains nine calories of energy in every gram, double the amount in a gram of carbohydrate or protein. *Efficient,* when used with *fat,* is a negative rather than a positive word. It's easier (more efficient) for the body to keep that fat around instead of using it quickly for energy, as it does carbohydrates or proteins.

The Journey of Fats Through the Bloodstream

Although fat can be used for fuel, the body turns up its hypothetical nose and opts, first, for glucose or fructose to meet its energy needs. Some parts of the body are very picky about this. The red blood cells and parts of the kidneys will not use any fuel except carbohydrates. The brain, by far the biggest consumer of energy in the body, strongly prefers glucose and will only grudgingly use fat for fuel if no glucose is around.

Now here is a little-known but essential fact. You recall that glucose can be converted to fat. The reverse is not true. Fat cannot be converted to glucose and used by the body for energy. Once the fat you eat is divvied up and the portion needed as raw material and the portion needed for fuel is allocated, all the rest is stored as fat. This is not an expensive biological process.

In fact, from an energy point of view, it's real cheap. Only 3 percent of the energy contained in fat is used up in processing fat for storage, so a full 97 percent is preserved to be deposited into the fat stores of your body.

Are you beginning to see why dietary fat is bad news? Fat is both calorically dense and efficiently stored. So if you want to get fat or stay fat, eat fat. It's not a bad way to shorten your life, either.

You would have to be living in a cave not to know that there is serious concern in the professional health community about the amount and type of fats in the American diet. Excessive fat intake is clearly linked to the development of heart disease and strokes. Fat is also seen as the culprit in some very serious forms of cancer. We have all been told to cut back on our intake of fat, especially saturated fats.

All right. Why all the fuss about *saturated fat*, the type that makes hamburgers juicy and chicken skin crisp and butter taste *so* good? Saturated fat is bad because of its effect on cholesterol levels.

Cholesterol is a category of blood lipids, and lipids are fats. There are two forms of cholesterol: *high-density lipoproteins* (HDLs) or "good" cholesterol and *low-density lipoproteins* (LDLs) or "bad" cholesterol. HDL cholesterol is carried out of the bloodstream for removal from the body, whereas LDL cholesterol is carried to the cells for use.

Cholesterol is a very important molecule in the body in the proper amounts, and the body tries very hard to regulate its level in the blood. For example, your liver can make cholesterol whenever it wants to, but it will shut down production when you eat foods that are high in dietary cholesterol to try to keep the blood level normal. Even the cells in the body help regulate cholesterol by creating special receptors that pull cholesterol out of the blood.

This is where saturated fat does its damage. It diminishes the production of these receptors, thus keeping more LDL cholesterol in the blood. And where does this excess cholesterol go? Unfortunately, it tends to get deposited in the lining of blood vessels, narrowing the passageways within them and eventually blocking them completely. When the blood vessels serving the heart get totally blocked, you have a heart attack.

Unsaturated fat does not have this effect. It can actually help lower LDL cholesterol levels. It may lower HDL levels as well, however, which you don't want. The best type of fat to eat is *monounsaturated fat*, the kind found in olive and canola oil. It also helps lower LDL cholesterol and does not seem to have a negative effect on HDL levels.

That's the fat story. Here's a brief summary to help you review.

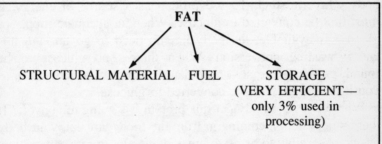

FAT

STRUCTURAL MATERIAL   FUEL   STORAGE
(VERY EFFICIENT—
only 3% used in
processing)

SATURATED: Diminishes receptors that pull cholesterol out of blood. Keeps LDLs high which deposits cholesterol in lining of blood vessels.

UNSATURATED: Lowers both HDLs and LDLs.

MONOSATURATED: Lowers only LDLs.

FACTS ABOUT PROTEIN

We now turn to the final nutrient, that marvelous, mystical substance that has played such a major role in the history of dieting, protein. At one time, early in the 1970s, high-protein diets were the rage. A few examples still exist today but most experts now feel that a diet too high in protein is not good for you because it puts a strain on the kidneys (as you will learn below).

Proteins, the building blocks of all of the organs and muscles of the body, are complex molecules made up of long chains of amino acids. There are twenty-two amino acids, only eight of which your body can't produce by itself and needs to get from dietary protein. So dietary protein is an essential raw material needed to build and repair and maintain your organs and muscles.

But what about protein as a fuel? Can the body use protein as a source of energy the way it uses carbohydrates and fats? Actually, the body prefers not to. Remember that glucose is the body's favorite fuel. To use protein as a source of energy, it must first be converted to glucose. When an adequate supply of glucose is available, the body has no need to go through this energy-wasting conversion. When there's no glucose to be found, protein is the next candidate in line for the job, since, as you'll recall, fat can't be converted to glucose.

Where does the body get this protein it's going to convert? If there's not enough coming in from the foods you eat, your body has no choice but to begin to break down and *use its own protein for fuel*. That means the body can survive only by removing protein from its own muscles and organs. People who are starving (or obsessively trying to lose weight on unbalanced diets) appear wasted for the very good reason that they are being eaten alive.

It can be dangerous to consume too little protein, especially when you're dieting and delivering less fuel to the body than it needs for maintenance and repair. (Clearly, children, teenagers, pregnant and nursing mothers, and those recovering from illness or trauma need even more protein than the rest of us, to build new tissue or repair damaged tissue.)

But what about too much protein? Is it a bad idea to eat too much? Modern nutritional thinking says yes.

When you eat proteins, they are broken down into amino acids before they enter the bloodstream. The body will first choose to use these amino acids for the physiological repair work we discussed above.

The remaining amino acids have one of two fates. They can be converted to glucose for fuel or converted to fat for fuel storage. Protein, like carbohydrates, can be converted to fat. Like carbohydrates, about 25 percent of the energy contained in protein is used up in this conversion. What makes too much protein dangerous, however, is the fact that amino acids are nitrogen-containing molecules, and excess nitrogen is a potentially toxic substance in the body. The conversion of amino acids to glucose or to fat requires that the nitrogen be removed from the amino acids and delivered to the kidneys for disposal.

Too much nitrogen damages the kidneys. The more protein you eat, the more nitrogen must be spun off the amino acids, and the more stress is put on the kidneys. For this reason, protein intake should be kept to a reasonable level. We'll discuss how much in Step 6. Protein is an essential nutrient, but it shouldn't be abused.

Let's go over the basic protein facts one last time. Below is a chart to help you review.

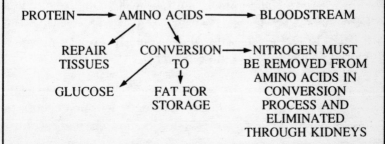

PROTEIN

Made of 22 amino acids. The body produces all but 8, which must be derived from diet.

USES OF PROTEIN

Raw material to build, maintain, or repair organs

Fuel—only in cases of severe dietary deprivation, when body converts its own protein to glucose if there is no other source

BREAKDOWN OF PROTEIN

PROTEIN → AMINO ACIDS → BLOODSTREAM

REPAIR TISSUES

CONVERSION TO

GLUCOSE

FAT FOR STORAGE

NITROGEN MUST BE REMOVED FROM AMINO ACIDS IN CONVERSION PROCESS AND ELIMINATED THROUGH KIDNEYS

That's the scoop on nutritional metabolism. Now you have accurate knowledge about what's going on inside you, and this empowers you to make some crucial decisions about your body and food. In Step 6, I'll enhance this knowledge by getting specific about what and how much to eat.

THE BENEFITS OF KNOWLEDGE ABOUT NUTRIENTS

The good thing about knowledge is that no one can wow you with pyrotechnics and sell you the Brooklyn Bridge. If you believe a bill of goods when you have the real facts at your disposal, you have no one to blame but yourself.

Remember that diet entrepreneurs view anyone with a weight problem as fair game. They will not hesitate to sell you absolutely worthless products or programs as long as they can get away with it (and make money). Have you ever been tempted by ads promising that you can burn fat effortlessly by taking a simple pill? Have you ever tried to lose ten pounds in one week on a high-protein, low-carbohydrate diet? I think we all have. When you allow yourself to be victimized this way, it contributes to your low self-esteem, especially after the plan or scheme doesn't work and you realize that you have been played for a sucker once again.

But that can't happen now. You have a working knowledge of the basic facts about metabolism, so you can never be victimized by charlatans and miracle-pill salesmen again.

Remember, knowledge is power. And with this power, you will begin to feel much better about yourself. So let's move on to more knowledge—and more power.

HOW FAT FUNCTIONS IN THE BODY: THE FAT CELL

If you have ever wondered what human fat tissue looks like, pay attention next time you are preparing a chicken because human fat looks a lot like chicken fat. At a microscopic level, fat is composed of billions of fat cells. A fat cell can be described as a little bag full of oil. There is not much to the cell because it really only serves one function—to store this oil until needed.

As a storage depot, the fat cell must be able to accommodate different storage demands. When the body's demand for the energy contained in fat goes up (like when you are dieting or starving), fat cells can shrink a thousandfold as they release their stored energy to the body. As the fat cells get smaller you get smaller, and you lose weight.

At some point, however, the fat cell begins to feel empty, eager to refill its depleted storage tank. The fat cell communicates this desire to fill up by making you hungry. Fat cells are notoriously disinterested in your desire to look slim. They are much more focused on their primary task, which is assuring your survival. And to this end, they do not want to be empty because this represents a terrible threat. They perceive dieting as a nasty trick to wipe out the organism. In their response to a famine in the land, they will try to motivate you to survive by eating.

And so you eat. And consume more fat. When so much fat is being consumed that the body can't use it all, and more fat needs to be stored, the fat cell can greatly increase in size. In fact, the fat cell can increase its storage capacity a thousandfold before it is full. In most cases, obesity represents an excess accumulation of fat storage, or larger fat cells.

But what happens when all of your fat cells are full and there is still demand for additional fat storage? At that point the body has no choice except to create new fat cells to hold the additional energy. Now here's the kicker. Once fat cells are created, they're there for good: They cannot be destroyed, even by the most rigorous dieting. So if you accumulate an excess number of fat cells, you are going to have a much more difficult time radically reducing the size of your body. As soon as this excessive number of fat cells shrinks to an unnaturally small size, they constantly will demand to be filled. That means you'll be hungry all the time.

Fat Cell Mania: Two Case Histories

Case #1: Julie. Julie came to me feeling desperate. She was determined to get back to her high school weight of 132 pounds. She had just been to a class reunion and felt humiliated when an old friend made a snide remark about the way she looked. Julie was 38 years old, stood 5 feet 6 inches tall, and weighed 188 pounds.

I introduced Julie to the concept of Fat Madness and helped her see that although she might feel better at a somewhat lower weight, her goal was unrealistic and her feelings of desperation were the result of years of cultural brainwashing. She began to understand that weight loss alone would not solve her problems with self-image and self-esteem.

Over a period of months, Julie and I worked to develop a lifestyle in which she enjoyed healthier eating and increased physical activity. As a consequence, her weight dropped to 146 pounds. She was able to maintain this weight without suffering constant hunger pangs or feeling deprived of the joys of eating. As for the snide remark at the class reunion, she learned to care less.

Let me take you inside Julie now—not inside her mind, which did a lot of changing, but inside her cells.

When Julie first came to me weighing 188, she was obese because of the *excess size of a normal number* of fat cells in her body, a condition known as *hypertrophic obesity*. When Julie lost weight, her fat cells reduced in size to a reasonable level.

They were not pushed to the point of being so small that they felt empty (achieving her original goal of 132 pounds would have caused this). But she could maintain the reasonable weight of 146 quite comfortably, eating a variety of foods and not feeling chronically hungry.

Case #2: Suzanne. Suzanne had a much more serious weight problem than Julie. (Note, please, that I am making a distinction between the weight problem itself, which is physical, and the Fat Madness problem they both shared, which is simultaneously physical, mental, and emotional.)

When I first saw Suzanne, she weighed 275 pounds. Fewer than eighteen months before, Suzanne had lost 111 pounds on a liquid diet over the course of just eight months. In the following ten months, she moved from that low of 155 to an all-time high of 275—nine pounds higher than she'd been before she started the liquid diet. She said the reason she gained back all of the weight was an uncontrollable feeling of hunger that was *never* satisfied by the 1,200-calorie maintenance diet her doctor prescribed for her.

As you can imagine, Suzanne was feeling miserable about herself when she came to see me. She was deeply ashamed about being so weak-willed, unable to resist the hunger that had made her gain back all of her weight.

I worked on Suzanne's Fat Madness problem first, explaining how her preoccupation with food and weight had kept her on a diet roller-coaster most of her life. This same problem had also caused her to give up when she couldn't maintain the unnaturally low weight she'd achieved and binged her way up to the highest weight she'd ever carried in her life. I then went on to explain how her initial intense hunger was a normal physiological consequence of her fat cell situation.

Suzanne's excess weight caused fat storage demands that not only filled up her existing fat cells but required the *creation of new fat cells* for more storage capacity, a condition known as *hyperplastic obesity*. When Suzanne reduced her weight drastically on the liquid diet, she forced her now excessively high number of fat cells to reduce below a reasonable size. They felt empty and sent out strong hunger signals until they filled back up.

The physiological hunger signal stopped when her fat cells got back up to a reasonable size. At this point, she probably weighed around 180 or 190 pounds. Why then did she gain back weight up to 275 pounds? After she reached 180 pounds, the physiological hunger eased. But Suzanne had broken her restraint and felt unable to stop herself. Her chronic problem with Fat Madness set her back on an inexorable path to 275.

Please understand that Julie and Suzanne, with two different types of obesity, will need different dieting goals and should have different weight loss expectations. I'll talk about this in detail in Step 4.

Julie and Suzanne have some other different qualities that they must consider. It's not always just a question of the size and number of fat cells in the body. Placement of the cells is also crucial. And here, biology is destiny.

Where the Fat Is Deposited
Makes a Difference in Your Shape

Men and women are shaped differently. Men putting on weight tend to deposit it around the abdomen and heart (a more dangerous type of fat deposition than the female variety). Females who are naturally more rounded at the breasts, hips, and buttocks, deposit their excess weight in these areas. This fact brings up some fundamental differences in the way specific fat cells store and release fat.

Scientists have only recently proven that all fat cells are not created equal. That's no big surprise to dieters. They've known this for years. Melanie is a classic example.

Case #3: Melanie. Melanie doesn't really have a serious weight problem. She does, however, have what she considers a very serious shape problem. Melanie's body looks like it belongs to two different people, one above the waist, one below. From the waist up, Melanie meets today's stringent standards of female beauty. There isn't an ounce of fat; her waist is thin and taut.

But from the waist down, her body looks like a "before" ad for a cellulite treatment clinic. Her hips flare from her waist, sheathed in massive deposits of subcutaneous fat. Her buttocks and thighs are puckered with loose fat.

By the time Melanie came to see me, she had tried everything short of plastic surgery to reduce her bottom half. She was a sucker for any spot-reducing diet, and of course, she always got the same frustrating results. Melanie would lose a modest amount of weight on her hips, but at a tremendous cost. She'd eat up what little fat she had on top, appearing anorexic and skeletal around her face and chest. Even her breasts got smaller. Her hips and thighs, however, stubbornly refused to cooperate.

I explained to Melanie that there were more crucial issues than the size of her hips. She, like Julie and Suzanne, had a lot of personal work to do to recover from Fat Madness. And following her recovery, the need for a radical solution to her body problem might not seem so important.

Then, I gave her the knowledge she lacked. Melanie was fighting biology, and biology was (as always) winning. Because in Melanie, as in all women, fat cells below the waist behave very differently from fat cells above the waist.

Evolution intended the female body to serve one primary purpose: to create, sustain, and support new life. Women clearly need more energy when they are nurturing a developing fetus or lactating, and this energy is supplied from an extra fat-storage depot below the waist. Some women, like Melanie, are more evolutionarily fit than others.

Obviously, since this fat has a special purpose, it can't be called into play to meet the day-to-day energy demands of the body. If it were, the body would run the risk of depleting this special store before it was needed for successful procreation. So this fat has special properties that allow it to resist releasing its fat stores into the bloodstream unless special hormonal conditions existed that signal pregnancy or lactation.

Melanie didn't care that she was beautifully built for childbearing. She just wanted to change her body shape. That, of course, is one of the only things she could never do. Remember, biology is destiny.

So let's turn now from the fat cell to the larger questions. Why are we built the way we are? Why does Melanie have to resign herself to culturally unfashionable hips while those who she envies (and there are many) have proportionate or, better yet, boylike hips and thighs? The answer is genetics.

Genetic Influences on Body Weight

You have control over a lot of elements in your weight control situation. You know that good nutrition and exercise are essential, and you know you're supposed to avoid fats as much as you can. Those are the facets of calories in/calories out that are within your personal take-charge realm.

But there are many things going on in your body that you're unaware of and can't control. We've all inherited a predilection for biochemical changes that happen on a microscopic level. These will ultimately decide whether it's easy or difficult for us to attain and maintain our culturally determined standard of physical attractiveness.

Genetics is responsible for about 25 to 35 percent of the various effects on the body that account for shape, size, and weight. What a strange convocation of decision makers are those tiny genes that sit two by two along your chromosomes! If you will harken back to Professor Mendel and his peas, you will recall that if you cross a pure dominant gene with a pure recessive gene, you will get two hybrids (AA + aa = Aa and aA) and the dominant trait will be the one that shows up. But in the next generation down, when you cross the hybrids, you will wind up with four possibilities (AA, aa, Aa, and aA).

If your mother is fat and your father is thin, but one of your dad's parents had a weight problem, you may wind up dieting your life away, trying desperately to overcome your genes. Studies have unequivocally proven that a tendency toward fatness can be inherited.

Genetic traits and the way they work have been closely monitored through studies of adopted children. Take genetically identical twins, for example. You can follow one particular trait and rate the role of environment vs. genetics and see which plays a larger part. An eminent bariatrician (a doctor who specializes in the treatment of obesity), Dr. Albert Stunkard, published an excellent paper in 1986 that proved the importance of genetics over environment—or nature over nurture—by comparing certain characteristics in each twin against those characteristics in both their biological and adoptive parents.

Even when the adoptive parents served fried doughnuts and cream cakes every day, the kids with a genetic tendency to be thin didn't bulk up to nearly the size of those children who had a genetic tendency to become fat. As it happens, 80 percent of the children of two obese parents become obese, as opposed to only 14 percent of the kids born to normal-weight parents, regardless of the eating habits of the adoptive parents who raised them.

In another study done by Drs. Bouchard and Miller in 1990, sets of twins were asked to gain and lose weight as their calories in and out were carefully counted. All the subjects ate and exercised exactly alike, and yet some of the twins gained or lost more. And they gained or lost just the way their twin did it!

What is the gene doing in the body that accounts for these differences? There are some interesting theories, although no one is quite sure. The first relates to an enzyme called lipoprotein-lipase that grabs fat from the blood and pulls it into the cell. The activity of this enzyme determines how many calories from the food you've consumed get pulled in to be stored as fat. This amount can vary greatly among people.

The genetic response in the body may actually be changing in America in response to some element in our diet. There is a lot of evidence showing that American kids are getting fatter in general, and that their overall metabolic rates are lower than those in children of other countries. It's thought that U.S. kids actually get to their excess fat more quickly because their propensity for fat deposition has become more efficient. In this case, efficiency is *not* what we want—we'd like to get the body to work really hard in order to have to store any of its fat.

This is a clear indication that a calorie isn't a calorie. Watching what you eat and measuring every slice of pie and every snack cracker will not necessarily control your body weight and shape. The way you deposit your nutrients as fat and the way someone else does varies widely due to your genetic ability to burn or store fat.

One unfortunate side effect of genetics is that we often try to compensate for undesirable genes with desperate behavior. Since the discovery of genetically engineered growth hormone, for example, many parents have requested this potentially dangerous compound for their genetically short children. We certainly don't have to look too hard to find evidence of desperate behavior about body weight. In fact, we don't have to look any farther than our supermarket checkout lines where the headlines of every rag mag proclaims that this or that celebrity suffers from bulimia or anorexia. There is no question that the epidemic of these deadly eating disorders has its roots in desperate attempts to alter genetic destiny.

Please remember that we are not entirely ruling out eating behavior as an important determinent of obesity. Eating junk food and excessive sugar and fats as well as eating great quantities will put weight on you. But because of genetic factors, some individuals will gain weight faster than others, and some will have more trouble losing weight if they are intentionally cutting back. You can control behavior; you can't play around with your genes. They're tailor-made for you, and you have to deal with them.

All About Setpoint

There's another scientific concept about hereditary factors in weight control that's been discussed in popular dieting books, and that is *setpoint*. It's often overlooked as an issue, possibly because it's so hard for many people to accept and use in a positive way. Setpoint is the thermodynamic rule of fat conservation in the body. This rule states that each person has his or her own natural range of weight (about ten pounds), under which it is hard to dip for any length of time.

The hypothalamus, the brain's thermostat, appears to be the controlling agent here. When you've been dieting so strenuously that your body is using up its fat stores, the hypothalamus reacts as it would if you were starving on a desert island. It begins to conserve energy very, very carefully, protecting the delicate mechanism that keeps us alive.

Everyone will remember Oprah Winfrey's battle with setpoint, which, unfortunately, she finally resolved by gaining back every one of the sixty-seven pounds she lost and a few more. Analyzing Oprah's struggle from the perspective of setpoint helps to explain exactly what happened to her. When Oprah achieved her fantasy goal of fitting into size ten jeans, she obviously dieted herself down to well below her setpoint. We can figure this out by looking at her killer maintenance program.

To stay a size ten, Oprah was forced to subsist on about 1,000 calories per day and was required to exercise vigorously for one or two hours per day. Most people would lose weight rapidly on the program that Oprah needed to follow just to maintain a weight loss. Obviously, she was fighting a war with her own biology, trying to maintain a weight well below her setpoint.

This does not, however, mean that Oprah has no possibility of maintaining a good healthy weight. All she has to do is understand setpoint and not set unreasonable goals for herself.

The difficulty for most chronic dieters in accepting the setpoint factor is kind of like the huge philosophical battle between predetermination and free will. For centuries, certain great thinkers have argued that we can't do anything much to change our lives—it's all fixed and written down in some great heavenly tome. Others have countered that man does and can change his destiny. All he has to do is be brave enough to break the mold, alter the pattern. To which the predestination folks say, sure, yeah, but that's all written down, too. You don't think you really had anything to do with changing your life.

Setpoint itself can be lowered with exercise, which minimizes the body's reaction to cutting back on calorie consumption.

Should you choose to maintain a weight lower than you really were born to carry, you are going to have to commit yourself to a lifelong, daily dose of strenuous physical exercise, which isn't really so bad. A lot of people find that they actually enjoy moving around a lot and continue to succeed at maintaining a healthy weight this way. (More about this in Step 6).

So, do you have free will? You always want to blame yourself for the plateaus you reach, either in your weight or your stamina. But understand that there are all these elements at work that minutely adjust your cells, your energy level, and your emotional ability to stay on course. You know there are times when you've adhered to a diet faithfully for weeks, and you haven't lost one ounce. And you despair. Well, don't. There are things beyond our power to control. Physiology is there, like a mountain. It changes, but slowly, over centuries of erosion and growth.

Life Events and Weight: Puberty, Pregnancy, and Aging

Before we move away from the physical factors that affect weight, we must briefly mention the times of your life when pounds quite naturally stick on you.

The first is at puberty, when young bodies are in enormous hormonal flux. The tendency to put on weight is most evident in girls, because they are busy getting ready to be women. In preparation for childbirth and nursing, the human female body begins to develop fatty tissue in the breasts, hips, buttocks, and thighs. Unfortunately, our society has deemed the rounded female body as something undesirable. No doubt, this is why eight out of ten female teenagers diet while only one out of four teenage boys do. It's also not surprising that the teenage years and early twenties, when the body is trying to grow the way nature says it should, are when most cases of anorexia and bulimia first present themselves. Anecdotal evidence indicates that the ages are stretching, though. Some children as young as seven or eight are obsessed with being fat. And some adults who are old enough to know better, already in their thirties and forties, still haven't grown out of their fear of fat and sometimes develop bulimia and anorexia at this late point in life.

The next natural spurt of fat deposition is at pregnancy. The body must store up its supply of fat in order to house and nourish new life. Physicians used to be bears about how much you couldn't gain (Remember the days when sixteen pounds was max?), which made most expectant mothers and many fathers, gaining sympathetically along with them, pretty crazy. The hormones are raging in the body at this juncture; and individual differences in pregnancy weight gain are legend. It is probably not a good idea to put on a great deal of weight very quickly, although there are extremely slight women who put on as much as one-third again their body weight. On the other hand, we have obese women who barely put on any weight at all during a pregnancy.

The problem comes after the baby is born. You have probably heard (maybe you've even said it yourself), "My body was never the same after the kids." Yes, well, except for movie stars and enormously wealthy people with personal trainers, we don't all have the determination to rehone all those stretched-out areas. Nor do we have the physical elasticity to rebound after our bodies have shifted shape so radically. It takes some women several years after a birth to lose the excess weight that came with carrying and bearing a child. Some never do. Nursing appears to make some difference for some women, no difference for others. Worrying probably makes the most difference, along with giving yourself permission, at last, no longer to be obsessed with dieting.

The third time of life that we naturally put on weight is during the aging process, starting about age fifty. Metabolism drops about 2 percent a decade, so it's easier to hold your weight five or ten pounds up from where you were at thirty or forty when you get older. And it's also a little extra protection for your bones, in case you should happen to fall, which you won't do as much if you're exercising every day and have developed balance and flexibility.

Some diseases associated with the aging process, such as certain cancers, will cause weight loss. But in the absence of illness, the tendency is for the body to increase its fat and lose muscle. The ratio of lean body mass to body fat goes down, and the amount of skeletal muscle and bone mass decreases too, particularly in women, who appear to be rounder and plumper, even if the scales say they haven't gained. Fat deposition as we get older tends to be on the trunk, which is the place you don't want it, but where it goes once the protective effects of hormone cycling disappear after menopause.

WORKING WITH YOUR NEW KNOWLEDGE

These are the biological facts you need to know for your Fat Madness Recovery Program. As you can see, there is a lot going on biologically that you can't control. Who can fight 2 million years of complex evolutionary changes? Look at it this way: Living organisms have been around a lot longer than the fashion industry. Viewed from this time frame, it's easy to understand how survival outweighs looks. Biology is reality.

It's okay if you can't accept these facts completely right now. It's enough to know that they are there for you, waiting to take their place in your lexicon of powerful tools to fight Fat Madness. Acceptance takes time, and it will come.

Before you can accept, you have to be able to let go. Let go of what, you ask. Oh, not too much. Just all of the insanity about your body weight and appearance that your culture and family and friends have fed you for your entire life.

In the following chapter, I'll explain exactly which psychological and emotional bonds you can break as we take apart some long-standing myths about your body image and weight maintenance.

Nutritional Metabolism Quiz

Test the knowledge you've gained in this chapter. If you don't get an A+ on this test, go back and review the sections you may be having trouble with.

1. The three main nutrients used by the body are _____, _____, and _____.

2. Proteins can be converted to fat but not to glucose.
   True_____ False_____

3. Complex carbohydrates cause blood glucose levels to peak and fall rapidly. True_____ False_____

4. Saturated fats raise blood cholesterol levels by:
   a. Increasing liver production of cholesterol
   b. Diminishing cell production of LDL receptors
   c. Raising HDL cholesterol levels
   d. All of the above

5. If an excess of 100 calories of fat is eaten, how many calories will be stored as fat? _____calories. What if an excess of 100 calories of carbohydrates is eaten? _____calories.

6. Proteins are long chains of _____ _____.

7. Glucose is the preferred fuel used by:
   a. The red blood cells
   b. Parts of the kidney
   c. The brain
   d. All of the above

8. Describe two advantages of eating complex carbohydrates.

_____

_____

9. You could live without eating any fat at all.
   True _____ False _____

10. Eaten in moderation, the best type of fat is:
    a. Monounsaturated
    b. Unsaturated
    c. Saturated

ANSWERS TO QUIZ:
1. Carbohydrates, proteins, and fats
2. False. Proteins can be converted to both fat and glucose.
3. False. Simple carbohydrates cause this.
4. Diminishing cell production of LDL receptors
5. 97 calories, 75 calories
6. Amino acids
7. All of the above
8. Stable blood glucose levels, and the fact that they are usually combined with other important nutrients
9. False. Fat is an essential nutrient.
10. Monounsaturated

Carbohydrates

1. Come in simple (short chain) and complex (long chain) forms
2. Are the preferred fuel of the body for immediate energy needs
3. May be stored as glycogen or fat
4. 25 percent of energy used up in conversion to fat
5. Complex carbohydrates deliver steady levels of glucose and nutrition

Fats

1. An essential nutrient and important building block
2. Most efficient form of energy storage
3. Contain 9 calories per gram vs. 4.5 for carbohydrates and protein
4. Cannot be converted to glucose for fuel
5. 97 percent of energy conserved for storage
6. Come in three forms: saturated, unsaturated, and monounsaturated
7. Monounsaturated best for controlling cholesterol levels

Proteins

1. Made up of chains of amino acids
2. Chief building blocks of muscles and organs
3. May be converted to both glucose and fat
4. Conversion uses up 25 percent of the energy in proteins
5. Conversion results in excess nitrogen, toxic to the kidneys

STEP 3: ACCEPT (ONE)

I Accept the Need to Let Go of Myths and False Hopes About My Body

Once, in the faraway land of Perfectbody, there lived a woman who feared greatly for her shape. She believed with all her heart that one cookie would make her fat forever. And so, though it turned her hair gray and her temperament sour, she restrained herself and refrained from eating the cookie.

One day, a slender snake curled around what appeared to any outsider to be her curvaceous leg (though *she* thought it might have been a discard from a piano company) and up her apparently normal-size stomach (which *she* viewed as stuffing for a pillowcase) to her arm, which was the only part of her anatomy of which she approved.

"Eat the cookie," the snake suggested. "I did, and look how thin I am."

"Oh, I couldn't," the woman protested. "I don't have your body. And I am a female. I wouldn't."

"Sure you would. Your best friend did, and your mother did, and [he lied] all those models on television did. Go on, live a little."

The woman took a breath and ate the cookie in two bites.

And she became horribly, grossly fat.

Not because she ate the cookie (she had not gained an ounce or a centimeter).

She became fat because she looked in the mirror and pronounced herself fat.

And her gray hair grew white and her sour temperament grew

monstrous, and she vowed (once again) that she would never eat the cookie.

You Are Your Own Myth-Maker

Isn't this myth ridiculous? Well, if it is, why aren't you laughing?

Because, even though you know it's a myth, you probably believe it with all your heart, and it hurts when you realize that you've done things and said things so similar during all your dieting years.

Now it's time to let go of all your old false hopes and self-defeating myths about your body.

- If I don't eat all day, then I can eat all night and not gain weight. WRONG.
- If I just taste while I'm cooking, it doesn't count. WRONG.
- If I lose twenty pounds before the class reunion, I'll have a great time; if I don't, I'll be miserable. BULL.
- If I eat one slice of that wedding cake, I'll burst out of my dress and everyone will laugh at me. UNTRUE.
- If I eat too much on my date, he'll be turned off and never ask me out again. RIDICULOUS.
- If I diet because my spouse/lover/mother/father wants me to "look better," I'll be really motivated to stick with it. BUNK.
- If I buy chips at the health food store instead of the supermarket, I can eat all I want because they're good for me. MISERABLE LIE.
- If I stop eating for five days, I can drop ten pounds and keep it off. TOTALLY WRONG.
- If I diet down to my perfect weight, my life will be perfect. IF YOU BELIEVE THAT, I'VE GOT A BRIDGE TO SELL YOU.

Why do we persist in holding onto our belief in the extraordinary statements above? And there are hundreds of others I could point to that are equally ingrained in us and equally wrong.

We generally acquire our beliefs, whether they are about ephemeral subjects such as politics and religion, or more concrete issues like health and fitness, from a combination of elements. First, we believe what we are taught to believe. Our most deeply held and inflexible beliefs have their roots in our childhood experiences at home and in school. Many people are hard-pressed when asked even to name these beliefs; they have become so rooted and integrated into our thinking that we hardly realize that they are beliefs, which makes them difficult to examine and modify. Many Fat Madness beliefs fall into this category. A good example of a bad belief: "It's attractive to be thin."

We are all so stuck on this belief that most of us feel it has to be fact, even gospel truth. Well, here's a little surprise. If you look at the whole world today, in the 1990s, you will find that the vast majority of cultures do not view thin women as the most attractive. Most cultures prefer that women be plump and curvaceous, especially below the waist. Aha! But wait. Before you decide to move to another country, have hope. Even the most deeply ingrained beliefs can be changed *if you want to change them*.

The second reason we believe what we believe is because of the media. We saw something on television or read something in a book or magazine that convinced us. And there are a lot of writers, producers, marketers, and advertisers out there who grew up learning the art of subtle and not-so-subtle persuasion and can now apply it to any field. When the advertisers turn their formidable talents to reinforcing and promoting beliefs we already hold as cherished and unquestioned, double whammy. This is clearly the case with our Fat Madness myths and beliefs about our weight and self-worth.

Finally, we also tend to believe just exactly what we want to believe. When you are involved in a minor altercation with another driver, you can bet you believe that you came to a dead stop at the four-way stop sign and the other guy jumped the gun. If your spouse is suddenly away every Thursday night at "office meetings," do you believe that piece of information when all evidence points to its falsehood? You bet you do. It's not that the spouse is the last to know about an affair; it's that the spouse doesn't *choose* to know for self-protective reasons.

This is also the case with the false hopes you may cherish about your body. It is vastly preferable to cling to a set of beliefs that could—possibly, maybe, if you stretch reality a little bit—come true than to sit down and look yourself square in the face, accept reality, and actually *do* something to change your situation.

A Killer Myth: Breaking the Body Into Parts

Jennifer is consumed with her belly. "The rest of me is really okay," she says, "but then I look in the mirror just before I go to bed and I see this mound of flesh hanging there with this weird puckered belly button, and I start to cry. It's always been terrible, but it's been much worse since my son was born three years ago. I do a hundred sit-ups a day and nothing helps. I just get a stomachache trying to hold my belly in all the time."

Lydia is obsessed with the hanging skin on her upper arms ("chicken skin," she calls it). And Maggi is embarrassed about the fact that her rear end ("bubble ass," she calls it) looks huge in the mirror when she's working out at the gym. Even Mark, who's a trim, athletic guy, is constantly checking out his love handles. When a woman touches him affectionately, he automatically feels uncomfortable, convinced she'll be turned off by those "gross hunks of flesh" below his ribs.

What we notice about these dissatisfied customers is that they believe that life has dealt them a lousy hand. If they could just rid themselves of one part of their body, all would be well. Seeing the body as a collection of parts rather than a whole is, obviously, a good way to ensure that you will never like your body. No matter how much weight you lose or how hard you exercise, this way of thinking guarantees that there will always be some part of your body that still needs fixing.

So the quest never ends, the task is never done, the goal is never reached. The body issue constantly replays itself, keeping us from ever achieving any peace of mind about what we look like. Why don't we ever come to the realization that this kind of thinking about the body is self-defeating and just let it go? The reason is that it is not only self-defeating, it is also self-supporting.

When you keep up the illusion that one body part is defective, you absolve yourself of the responsibility of working on the whole individual. If you're ashamed of one part of you, so ashamed that you can't imagine how other people can bear to look at it, then you are too busy sticking your head (or some other body part) in the sand to devote the proper amount of time and energy to working on the things you really can change. And believe me, you *can* do something positive about your attitude, your mind, your emotions—the elements other than your body that make you an individual.

"I can't stand that critical point in a relationship when I'm finally ready to have sex with a man," Abbey told me at one of our Fat Madness workshops. "I know when I take off my clothes that he's going to see how ugly my thighs are and be totally turned off. When I start getting close to somebody, the first thing I do is run back to the gym and start some spot reduction. Then I wait and dread the inevitable moment coming. Sometimes I break off the relationship just before, because I can't stand the thought of any man looking at my thighs."

What is this? Some perverse form of safe sex? Avoiding intimacy because of thigh shape and size? Well, maybe it didn't start off that way, but now fear of a body part serves the function of avoiding intimacy. As long as Abbey is concentrating on her thighs, she gets to avoid all of the issues that really underlie her fears of sex.

Is Abbey unusual? Not at all. Most of us have some part of us that we find unsightly. Maybe it's thick ankles or thin lips or even a birthmark in an odd spot. And our preoccupation with this is completely out of proportion to reality. Sometimes it directly interferes with our social or occupational growth. We would be amazed to find, however, that the people around us barely notice our knees or our noses. They may be too busy worrying about their own knees or noses. What we believe to be essential to our beauty, our completeness, and our desirability rarely has much to do with the reasons that other people like us, lust after us, or are indifferent to our charms.

You know this deep down inside, just as you now know the hard, cold nutritional information that ought to be guiding your eating behavior. It isn't possible, however, for you to use the facts at your disposal when your mind is cluttered with old beliefs, myths, and false hopes that contradict the truth.

If You Know What You Know, Then Why Do You Believe in Fairy Tales?

You have a vast body of knowledge about your genetic givens, your cultural adaptation to eating, and the biochemical processes that go on in the body. But seriously, folks, have the facts you learned in Step 2 caused you to make any really serious changes in the way you are currently behaving around your refrigerator?

The truth, you must admit, is that you stand in awe before the kitchen cabinets, peering through their open doors like Tiny Tim regarding the Christmas goose that miraculously appeared on his poor dining table, afraid to touch it lest it vanish like the rest of his dreams. You are totally baffled by the bounty around you, realizing that you still crave foods that you think you shouldn't have and don't have the slightest inclination for foods you've always believed to be acceptable (carrots and celery lead the dull and tasteless list).

You still wander in a trance down the aisles of the supermarket and into your own head as you consider the pasta, the potatoes, the bread. You repeat, like a mantra, all the information you had at your fingertips from Step 2. Complex carbohydrates are great; watch out for hidden fats; you can eat a cookie and not go to hell. You understand exactly what kind of food you're looking at and how it will affect you, inside and out.

But you do it anyway. You still walk past the potatoes and bread, because you see them as albatrosses around your hips, although you now know the truth. You still accept the slice of salami offered at the deli counter as you ponder whether your belly can actually do without the creamed cabbage salad and select the feta cheese instead. You belittle the influence of the salami in your war with your body because it's just a slice, you're standing up to eat it, it's not coming home with you, and anyhow, you can consume samples handed out in the supermarket because they don't count.

Isn't this ridiculous? And yet, we all do it. We all believe what we choose to believe, even if it's wrong and we know (or have been told by experts) what's right.

Myths Die Hard

The road from myth to reality is a slow and difficult one. It is the ultimate one-step-forward-two-steps-back experience. We cling to myths because they are reassuring and emotionally useful, allowing us the comfort of sticking with the past that has worked for us over and over, even if it has worked badly.

The new is unknown; this makes it untried and even dangerous. The new also sounds unpalatable (*not* dieting? *not* worrying about accumulating pounds?) and even impossible, so it seems pointless to try it just to be frustrated again.

Myths are a matter of personal creation, but they come from somewhere. Society has its own myths, which we'll explore in a minute, but we all have our own particular manner of transcribing those group myths for ourselves. What works for your best friend doesn't necessarily do a thing for you. For some, the food and body myths must be wildly imaginative and beyond the realm of possibility. For others, they must be allied to the truth, but not the truth. And others mix and match their myths, believing one thing one day and another thing another day, depending on what they really crave and what's available.

If It's Close to Your Mouth, You'll Eat It

Foods and eating experiences of childhood and the memories they evoke have a great deal to do with what you come to believe about weight and diet and how you eat as an adult. A person who grew up in a household where mayonnaise was slathered on everything from tunafish to guacamole, will tend to ignore the fact that mayonnaise is a high-fat food. Those who grew up to believe that salads are good for you will continue to chow down on greasy croutons and blue cheese dressing at every salad bar, and then wonder why the weight isn't falling off.

Someone who got milk and cookies for a snack every day after school has an emotional allegiance to those foods, particularly in combination. Childhood habits create their own myths. The myth that food soothes the emotions and should be a reward for good behavior is a particularly powerful one, enduring despite the thousands of adult experiences that teach you otherwise. How successful is it to binge on milk and cookies to calm your frazzled nerves when the eating experience itself creates remorse, guilt, and self-hate?

The family creates many potent eating myths. When the family does something together, whether it's going to church or consuming pints of ice cream every Saturday night, it is sanctioned behavior. Your mother may have talked about the fact that it was wicked to eat the remains of the Christmas candy before lunch on New Year's Day, but if she did it, and allowed you to do it, then by gum, it had family value.

Because our parents' generation was for the most part unaware of the destructive nature of cyclic overeating and dieting, we often saw these behaviors, which we know today are ill-advised and compulsive. And the media, unfortunately, is stuck in the dieting mentality of the last generation. Think about the elderly women in the television commercial regarding the beautiful model emerging from her makeup trailer in a silver lamé gown, clutching a can of diet soda. "We better start drinking

Diet Pepsi!'' one normal-sized seventy-year-old says to another, enviously regarding the smashingly sexy girl.

Is she kidding? Is that soda going to take off thirty of her pounds and fifty of her years? Not on your life. But the commercial implies that it will, and, on some level, we believe it.

If we know our enemy and look him smack in the eye, we can begin to gather our inner forces and outer armor and learn what makes him so fearsome. He can teach us his strengths and we can sap him of his energy by absorbing those brave qualities. (Remember the ancient tribal warriors who ate their foes in order to consume their fighting spirit?)

In this case, the enemy is the collection of false ideas about and your eating habits that you've accumulated over the years. Let's start identifying some of the myths that hamper us and get right down to the ruthless and concrete task of accepting ourselves as we are and altering only what may be detrimental to our physical health, longevity, sense of self-worth and well-being.

When it comes to weight loss and maintenance, you have to be a realist. You must identify the myths and false ideas that can set you up for failure in your weight-control efforts. The following quiz will bring you back to the wishes and fantasies so deeply embedded in your thinking about your body. Analyze your thoughts honestly and with care, to explore how Fat Madness has affected you.

Weight and Body History Quiz

Here are ten core myths and false hopes typically seen in cases of Fat Madness. Read each myth and then score it on the following scale:

Strongly agree:	3 points
Generally agree:	2 points
No opinion:	1 point
Disagree:	0 points

Be honest with yourself! The answers to this quiz are totally private, between you and yourself. Don't answer what you think you should believe, just put down what you do believe.

1. I'm fat because I eat for emotional reasons. Score _____
2. Losing weight requires a special program. Score _____
3. When I lose weight, I'll look great. Score _____
4. I can totally reshape my body. Score _____
5. (Women) I must wear a size 10 or less. Score _____
   (Men) I must have a size 34 waist or less. Score _____
6. I'm fat because I cannot resist fattening food. Score _____
7. My sex life will be better when I lose weight. Score _____
8. I can't be seen in a bathing suit. Score _____
9. I must lose weight quickly. Score _____
10. I could not possibly learn to live with my body Score _____
as it is right now.

How did you score? The myths that scored a three are going to need your undivided attention, twos will need some work; the ones and zeros are not going to be problems for you.

I want you to take this quiz and put it aside for a while. At the end of this chapter, after you've understood a little more about how these myths came to play a part in your life and in the lives of most of the people you know, I'll explore some of the reasons that you may have answered the way you did and give you some food for thought about how these myths can sabotage your efforts for sensible and lasting weight control. (Don't worry—food for thought isn't fattening.)

Right now, it's time to look back and discover the roots of the myths. They didn't arrive fully blown in your head; they were around for centuries. Our fixation with weight and dieting is a long-standing and distinguished madness.

The History of Fat Madness

Plumbing the depths of your past for clues is essential to gain easier acceptance of yourself. You have to stop blaming yourself for believing the things you've grown up believing, and you also have to realize where these credos came from.

There is a long international tradition of obsession about weight. In the Renaissance, royalty used to stuff themselves at feast time, then hie themselves to a country retreat, which we would today term a spa, for purges and high colonics to get rid of all the excess poundage. In the following centuries, all you have to do is look at a period costume book for a clue to craziness about weight. Waists were pulled in with corsets of whalebone, yanked to such constrictive proportions that many ribs were broken and hopes for conception and childbearing dashed. Women hid in closets to eat, then hid in water closets to purge themselves. They had to look a certain way for their fathers, for their eligibility as brides, and for their social station.

History abounds with stories and anecdotes about beauty being tied to femininity. And what do we consider feminine? Eating small meals is polite and dainty. There are a lot of small, delicate, charming words that show up in the Thesaurus as synonymous with feminine, and as you well know, the pen is mightier than the sword. Words mean a lot, and our connotations of *woman* that come down to us through the centuries are very heavily loaded with expectations of how a woman is supposed to look—and eat.

Of course, the excessive quest for thinness is ultimately self-defeating. Looking at the psychological studies done on body image, we can see that women's concerns about what other people think of them affects behavior drastically.

Let us go back and look at fashion in the first two decades of the twentieth century in America. The world had just been stunned by the women's movement, and suffragettes, though often mocked, were a profound influence on the average housewife. There were incredibly brave souls like Margaret Sanger, who preached that a woman would never be completely free until she had sexual autonomy; there were Susan B. Anthony, Lucretia Mott, and Elizabeth Cady Stanton, who marched so that women could vote for their elected officials; and Jane Adams, who took on housing and public sanitation for the poor. Did these women have time to worry about their figures? Certainly not.

Just look at what women were wearing in the 1920s. Off came the bustles, up came the hems. The curvaceous female looked a little awkward in the straight-line, no-nonsense dresses that seemed to ask, "Why can't a woman look more like a man?" Flat was in. Fat was out.

Marlene Dietrich and Katharine Hepburn became stars in the following decade, and fashion changed again. The androgenous Dietrich seduced in a tuxedo, and was considered a cagey, slightly dangerous female. Hepburn, all spit and polish and terribly self-assured, swaggered in pants better than any man who played opposite her. She was so smart, you can almost see her thinking her way in and out of situations on camera.

The correlation of fashion and thinness to our perception of women's competence and brilliance has persisted to the present day. Statistical studies show that when there are more women in the professional workforce, the media shows us thinner models. Women themselves seem to feel that not looking round and juicy is one of the criteria for getting a good white-collar job.

Remember all those man-tailored suits with ties that women were supposed to wear to the office in the early 1980s? And what do you know? They've recently come back!

This phenomenon has been studied by several noted modern-day researchers such as Rodin in 1984, and Striegel-Moore, Silberstein and Rodin in 1986. Women were asked to fill out self-esteem questionnaires where topics ranged from whether they felt their fathers thought they were smart or pretty to whether they liked their bodies. Time after time, it was clear that women who wanted to pursue traditionally male careers thought they should be thinner. The dominant feelings of perfectionism, desire to achieve academically or professionally, negative self-image, and extreme focus on the body came through in all these women.

Thinness, after a while, wasn't enough. Not only did society and the media decide how much people ought to weigh, they had the audacity to say where the weight was supposed to go. In the late 1960s, Jane Fonda and others became fitness nuts and developed muscles. Working out became a way of self-punishment rather than a journey toward health. If you didn't have sculpted pecs and not a drop of cellulite, it didn't matter if you weighed 110.

We've pinned this whole thing on women, but in fact, it affects all of us. Elementary school children were shown photos of all kinds of kids and asked which ones they'd like to be friends with. The preferences in all classes, races, and ethnic groups (except for the Jewish sampling, where the cultural ideal is not particularly svelte) were for thin kids. Even kids in wheelchairs and kids without one hand were picked before the obese children!

We are intensely prejudiced against fat people. It happens to be the case that those who are over the desirable weight range for their height do have more trouble getting jobs and getting ahead in their careers. And of course, this prejudice is genderless, affecting men as much as women. There are now guys who monitor everything they eat and go crazy with exercise. The advent of "roid rage" is a truly scary one—certain steroid users even deprive themselves of water in order to achieve a perfect form. Did you know that the current standard for male models is a size twenty-eight waist? Men are currently seeking counseling just like their female cohorts for their predilection to both anorexia and bulimia.

You Are Susceptible to the Forces Around You

When you examine your reactions to the issues on our Weight and Body History Quiz, you may be shocked to discover how much of your thinking is consolidated around the propaganda you see every day, which you feel doesn't affect you.

Sometimes pride stands in the way of admitting that we are indeed susceptible to influences such as television commercials and articles in newspapers and magazines. In my experience with participants in my Fat Madness workshops, as well as my talks with friends, colleagues, and family, I would say that everyone is affected to some degree. Unless you go through some process of letting go in order to handle these myths, you will never be able to fully accept the need for a rational program of lifetime weight maintenance. In order to achieve peace of mind, which is better than any fantasy, you will ultimately have to give up on the ideal body image and perfect weight the media has concocted for you and accept the goals that you can actually accomplish.

What Can We Do About This Obsession?

The craziness that surrounds food and eating has been adversely affecting you since you were a child. What can you do to change it? No, you can't march on Washington to protest the way the media has used and abused you. You can't write your congressman, because she or he undoubtedly has the same mentality you do about what food means. But you *can* act as an individual. You can choose to undo the damage by creating a way not to be brainwashed anymore. You know as well as I do that your fears and humiliation and embarrassment and sense of failure are triggered by the unique and perverse master plan created by the media. You can rise above it by letting go of it.

Think about marketing. Everything you see and touch from a slice of cheese to an insurance policy is marketed. Somebody out there (lots of somebodies, actually, since all decisions these days are made by focus groups) decided to induce in you and your mother and neighbor and everyone else with access to a newspaper, magazine, radio, or television, a sense of acute dissatisfaction with your own life. If you only had a yellower piece of cheese or an insurance policy that covered you *even* for acts of God, you would be happy. If you only used a little more of that mascara and this lipstick, surely you would be the spitting image of Michelle Pfeiffer. As soon as you go out and get a pair of those terrific-fitting shorts like the Olympic athletes wear, you'll be able to swim, dive, vault, and be built like those teenage gods and goddesses.

Desire leads to consumption, which leads to increased dissatisfaction when the product doesn't deliver. But that's okay, because if we bought the permanently right color shirts this year, we wouldn't buy any next year. Fashions must change so we can want some more. If we achieve the current ideal, then the marketing poobahs will give us a new one and new accoutrements to go with it.

This isn't just a jaded view of the way the world turns. It's the truth, and you can ask any marketing person. But there's something else going on, which I have to admit is not all bad. This is that the desire to be lean and mean is a response to increasing health awareness in America.

We of the United States of Physical and Mental Consciousness try—oh so hard do we try—to eat and exercise right because it's good for us. It will make us look better, feel better, live longer, and—here's the kicker—be phenomenally attractive to the opposite sex.

Marketers zero in on our need for the things that will make us look just like the people in the advertisements wearing that gel-activated running shoe or that sweat-wicked-away Capilene singlet. And if the twenty-one-year-old skinny, lithe model doesn't turn us on, they'll recast the ad with fifteen-year-olds, whose bodies are even farther away from our own and therefore less attainable.

Cultural brainwashing is about money. The perfect image we've grown up with of the way we'd like to see ourselves is all tied up with the need to spend money on things that will change us irrevocably. Until we stop buying into the buying system, until we believe that we're basically okay on our own and that we are in this body for this life, nothing will change.

Myth Reduction

Earlier in this chapter, you took a quiz. Your answers came from deep within you. They are so close to you right now that you couldn't possibly respond to them in any other way. In time, however, after you've blown apart your preconceived notions, your opinions will change. Now that you are aware of their long and insidious tradition, you can examine these myths, which are so universal, we hardly even think anymore about where they came from. I'm going to take each one of them apart so that you can see their foibles and fallacies.

1. I'm fat because I eat for emotional reasons. This is a powerful myth in our culture. More and more desperate dieters have been showing up in my practice convinced that they will find the solution to their chronic cyclic weight problem if they can uncover and work through problems from their past. They believe that the emotional residue from past traumatic events has fostered their patterns of compulsive overeating, which of course has been responsible for the regain of all that weight they lost many times over on many "successful" diets.

This myth comes from the veteran dieters' conviction that there is an irresistible force causing them to gain back all of the weight they lose. I agree. I call that irresistible force Fat Madness. We've all been subject to the shared brainwashing that tells us that if you have a weight problem, there is something wrong with you. And feeling that you're defective in this essential way shatters your self-esteem and programs you to fail.

I do not agree, however, that deeply rooted personal psychological problems and past traumas are the deeper cause of overeating and regaining lost weight.

First, it has been clearly documented that overweight people are not more psychologically disturbed than normal weight and thin people. Some studies have even reported that the overweight people are somewhat better adjusted to life and its hardships than others. This would argue against a lengthy and often painful psychological exploration of your past in order to get rid of your long-term weight control problem.

This myth is harmful as well as being undocumentable. It hurts us because it holds out the promise of a magic solution or cure for what is really a chronic, relapsing, addictive pattern of behavior. If you're busy lounging on a shrink's couch exploring past traumas and painful events, you are distracted from the very challenging and concrete behavioral and cognitive tasks that need your undivided attention right now.

This is not to say that there is never a place for psychotherapy in the treatment of chronic weight control problems. Sometimes it can help as a support in an ongoing recovery program. But let's not cop out and generalize about all people who overeat having deeply rooted psychological problems. It's a myth that needs to be blown apart.

2. Losing weight requires a special program. This myth is perpetuated by the marketing forces behind the big diet programs, and it can be a very expensive one to believe in. One of my patients, Marjorie, estimates that she has spent over $40,000 on weight loss programs in her life and now weighs more than she ever did. How much have you spent?

This myth is sustained by the low self-esteem of Fat Madness victims. It forces chronic dieters to seek out one program or product after another, hoping that the next will be the magic pill, the perfect fix. It doesn't touch the true source of their inability to sustain a weight loss. Remember, it's not the diet, it's the dieter.

Weight-loss programs and products, just like psychotherapy, can sometimes be helpful if they aren't seen as a panacea. After all, we've agreed that weight loss requires deprivation, and people often need help coping with this uncomfortable physiological state. (We will discuss the pros and cons of the various weight loss programs and products in Step 5). Remember, though, that no program or plan will ever do the work for you that you have to do for yourself.

3. When I lose weight, I'll look great. Our cultural bias toward thinness gives us the impression that when we lose weight, everyone will think we look better. But will we really look great? Our standards of attractiveness are set by the media and go well beyond body weight. The right shape, the right height, and the right face we see on billboards, in print ads, and on television are the result of painstaking marketing searches for certain genetically endowed individuals. Marketers have created our myth of beauty from the look that they deem right, so we deem it right, too.

I hate to see how much emotional energy dieters devote to the pursuit of beauty, especially because they are invariably disappointed with the results. Faces are not reformed, breasts do not grow, muscles do not magically appear when pounds drop off. Sure, dieters know this. But the pursuit of weight loss is so all-encompassing, the goal so challenging and demanding, that they begin to mix up the beauty myth with the weight-loss myth. By confusing the two, they set themselves up for disappointment and failure. And then, in a what-the-hell-nothing-matters-anyway binge, they dive right off their maintenance program and back to their addictive behaviors.

4. I can totally reshape my body. A corollary to the previous myth is the belief that with the right program and enough effort, the body that God gave you can be totally reshaped to conform to some media-generated standard. This myth has launched very lucrative spot reduction and cellulite treatment programs.

How many times have you heard an exercise instructor tell you, "Today, ladies, we are going to work on those troublesome thighs"? Do you know that a certain television star has made tens of millions of dollars hawking an exercise machine to tone up and slim down women's thighs? Did you buy one? Did it work? Which closet is it stored in now?

Most people know that spot reduction is impossible, but they don't want to believe it. Let me tell you about the study on tennis players.

Some scientists decided to look at the right forearm on right-handed tennis players to see whether selectively exercising one particular muscle group would result in a total decrease of fat around those muscles.

As you know, tennis is basically a one-handed game. If you're a righty, and you're a pro tennis player, your right forearm muscles are incredibly more developed than your left (and vice versa). So it was no surprise when the scientists discovered that, yes indeed, the muscles of the right forearm were much larger and stronger than those of the left. But—here's the interesting part, folks—the thicknesss of the fat just below the skin was *exactly the same* in both arms. This proved that no matter how hard a particular group of muscles is exercised, there's no selective loss of fat in the vicinity of that muscle group. All those promises of a rock-hard, washboard tummy from a hundred sit-ups a day are false.

Fat is lost from the entire body mass, no matter what part of the body you are exercising. If you have two inches of fat stored above your abdominal muscles, then just exercising those muscles without losing total body fat will only result in larger, firmer muscles hidden below that same two inches of fat. And as we discussed in Step 2, some fat resists any and all change, especially fat below the waist in women. Who ever said life was fair or fat was reasonable?

Let's move on to the controversial issue of cellulite. I'm delighted to see that people who attend my Fat Madness seminars have caught onto the fact that fat is fat. Cellulite is not some special or unique tissue, it is simply fat. The particular puckering look of cellulite comes from the connective tissue that surrounds the fat. No exercise, wrap, electrical stimulation, lotion, or potion will get rid of cellulite, so save your money.

I am not saying that exercise is fruitless. Working out and doing some weight training can reshape your body *within limits*. And you need to learn to accept these limits and make your peace with them.

5. *(Women) I must wear a size 10 or less./(Men) I must have a size 34 waist or less.* How do we define dieting success? Are people really satisfied to get down to a weight within the ideal body weight range? No way.

Most people who diet in our society are *already* within the ideal body-weight range. If about 21 percent of Americans are overweight and 47 percent of women and 24 percent of men are dieting, then the numbers speak for themselves. Fat madness makes acceptable weights unacceptable.

This particular myth shows how irrational we get when we set weight-loss goals. I always get a laugh of recognition in my seminars when I predict that I can guess the weight-loss goals of every woman in the audience. I say, "If you are between 5 feet 5 inches and 6 feet you want to weigh between 120 and 130 pounds. From 5 feet to 5 feet 5 inches, 110 to 120 pounds are the magic numbers." Note that word *magic*? It's so appropriate, because we invest these numbers with totally magical properties. These weights, like the size 6 or 8 dress or 34 pant size, will deliver success, happiness and beauty.

Magic numbers and sizes are killers. They are goals that set you up for failure since they are usually unattainable and very rarely maintainable. Even when you succeed in the very difficult task of losing some weight, the deeply felt desire to always do more, to attain an unattainable goal, will still make you feel like a failure.

6. I'm fat because I cannot resist fattening food. This myth has a long and glorious history. Years ago psychologists came up with the idea that the difference between fat and thin people was how they responded to the sights, smells, and tastes of food. These external cues were supposed to get fat people all excited, whereas the thinnies supposedly resisted overeating without effort because they only responded to their internal cues of hunger.

What a crock! The fact is that most people respond to external cues and will eat, even when not hungry, when they see, smell, or taste a tempting array of goodies.

If you subscribe to this damaging myth, you'll really be hard on yourself whenever you deviate from the set diet plan, and you decide you're a weakling and a slob. How could you be so stupid as to break down and eat the quarter pounder with cheese and large fries? How could you not, every once in a while?

You are human, and like all humans, fat and thin, you respond to the taste, sight, and smell of food. The danger in believing this myth is that you start beating yourself up every time you jump off the wagon. But you *will* go off your diet every once in a while. You're expected to. No one should pressure themselves never to deviate from a diet. How should you handle this?

In Step 5, I am going to suggest that those of you who choose to lose weight try to comply as closely as possible with a weight loss eating plan, but if you do deviate, not to overreact and abandon the whole program.

7. *My sex life will be better when I lose weight.* This one can really twist you around. Let me illustrate with a case history.

When Mary started her diet, she had a lot of fantasies about how her life would change when she lost weight. One of her fondest dreams was that losing weight would revitalize her nearly nonexistent sexual relationship with her husband, Don.

Mary and Don had been married for fourteen years. They'd had a pretty good sex life until after the birth of their second child seven years before. Mary just hadn't been able to regain her pre-pregnancy shape. So now, she was banking on weight loss as the key factor in getting the heat back in her sex life. She firmly believed that if she was thin, she could raise her husband's libido back to where it had been when he first married her.

Mary starved herself and managed to get back down to a size 8. Don told her she looked great and he was really thrilled. But the libido meter barely budged. Mary was shattered. Finally, she and Don went to see a marriage counselor and eventually determined that his loss of sexual vigor was due to a number of things, and Mary's figure wasn't one of them. He'd had some major setbacks in his career, and these had put him into a chronic depression and damaged his self-esteem. Mary and Don were able to work on revitalizing their sex life with mutual understanding and compassion. However, by that time, Mary had gained back most of her lost weight.

You see, rather than being awakened to a new realization that Don's problems—not her body—were the cause of their sexual misunderstandings, she was bitterly disappointed that her sacrifice and starvation hadn't affected her husband in the least. So she started overeating again and stopped exercising. She totally bought into the myth that good sex between people depends on physical appearance. This hurt her, and it hurt her marriage. And it can hurt you, if you don't let go of this destructive false idea.

8. *I can't be seen in a bathing suit.* Life is not a rehearsal for the real thing. Life does not begin after weight loss. It is going on before, during, and after. If you wait around to be seen, to do something you love, to go to places you enjoy, you are wasting your time and your life. But this is a typical self-defeating myth in Fat Madness. It's based in the notion that what other people think about us is more important than what we think about ourselves.

Charlene loves the beach, especially the feeling of sitting at the water's edge and letting the waves crash over her body. Charlene goes to the beach with her family, but she hasn't been in the water in three years because she's too ashamed to be seen in a bathing suit. So she goes to the beach in long shorts and a loose top and enviously watches her family frolic in the surf.

This was the first myth that Charlene and I tackled when she came to see me. What would happen, I asked, if people saw her in a bathing suit? "They'd be turned off," she stated. "They'd make comments."

"And then," I asked, "then what would happen?"

"I don't know," she said, "I never really thought about it. I guess nothing."

Exactly. Nothing would happen. Yet we fear that other people's own Fat Madness and their need to pick apart everyone else's body is important in our lives. It keeps us on tenterhooks, always waiting for the day when that socially acceptable body arrives so we can start living.

You need to rid yourself of this myth before you even consider the issue of needing to lose weight. It can defeat you before you start. Or, if it is your source of motivation to lose those pounds, it can act as a setup for regaining your lost weight. Because in our harsh and judgmental society, like it or not, unless we resemble those anorexic fashion ads, there's always going to be one dodo on the beach who thinks it's a real hoot to criticize the way we look. Because she probably hates the way she looks!

9. I must lose weight quickly. "Lose 30 Pounds by the Summer," the ads blare. Pretty appealing, huh? I hope you know by now that this is also pretty dangerous.

Rapid weight loss can cause a host of medical problems, not the least of which is gallbladder disease (more on this in Step 4). The desire to lose weight rapidly also causes a host of emotional problems that can make you want to give up on your diet and exercise program.

How many times have you stepped on the scale during a diet and your sense of cause and effect goes out the bathroom window? Well, when you step on the scale during a diet wishing with all your might that it will tell you that you've lost four or five pounds when you are only supposed to have lost one pound, this is magical thinking. It has no basis in logic.

The only way you can lose lots of pounds in a short period of time is by dropping some water weight. Losing water weight is only temporary. Those same four or five pounds can be regained in one day. Sound familiar? Does a five-pound weight gain during a diet make you want to give up? Sure it does.

Fat Madness causes you to put such a huge premium on weight loss that it becomes extremely difficult to accept the natural pace of the body's energy-balancing mechanisms. You expect the body to drop eight months of weight gain in only eight weeks. You know it can't work that way.

When you subscribe to the myth that you must lose weight quickly, you are setting yourself up for either physical complications from radical dieting or emotional disappointments from magical thinking. This is not the way to start a lifetime program of intelligent and successful weight management.

10. I could not possibly learn to live with my body as it is right now. In Step 4 you are going to be asked to make a very important decision. You are going to decide if it makes more sense for you to lose weight or to stay at your current weight and work on a healthier physical and emotional lifestyle. This is where Fat Madness really rears its ugly head. Listen to this telling quotation: "There are days where I hate my body. Like when I am doing a runway show and everyone else is a toothpick and I feel like a big moose. Or when I am trying on a swimsuit in fluorescent lights with those three-way mirrors—you know how it is.''

Who said that? Was it Queen Elizabeth? Was it a giant Russian weight lifter? Wrong. The quote is from none other than Cindy Crawford. If this woman doesn't love and totally accept her body the way it is, what chance do *you* have?

When you are in the grips of Fat Madness, this myth is a reality. The marketers and image makers out there (the ones who created Cindy Crawford) are banking on you not accepting your body, no matter what you weigh.

You must beat this myth. There will be no serenity, no peace of mind, and no final resolution of your food and body issue until you do. The later steps of the Fat Madness Recovery Program will address this issue head-on. But at this point I just want you to consider the possibility that you can learn to accept and love your body as it is. This is really possible. And you do not have to be bone-thin to do it.

So let go. Loosen the grip of this myth before you move on to important decisions and choices about weight loss.

Now that you have identified the myths and false hopes that have been keeping you from handling the way you feel about food and your body, you're on your way.

The Myth Called Euphoria

There is one myth bigger than all the others. It is the myth called *constant happiness*. Someday, if I try hard enough, if I look good enough, if I earn enough money, I will have constant happiness. There will be no little blips of dissatisfaction along the way—just perfection.

You know the corollary myth to this one: the one that promotes the false belief that you can be euphoric if you diet and succeed. The reason this myth falls apart is that if you are preoccupied with perfection, you'll never achieve the success you're looking for. The least little fall from grace—eating the cookie in Perfectbody—takes away happiness.

We have been brought up to believe that happiness is only winning the gold; silver is a consolation prize, and bronze is as bad as coming in last.

Yet, when you accept that this constant euphoria isn't around anyone's corner—not yours or any of the models on television—you will be much happier. You can suffer the bad stuff when you gain distance and perspective from it and learn how to cope with it. In fact, the only constant we can ever hope for is peace of mind and contentment.

Here's what to do: Don't strive for perfect bliss, perfect euphoria, or constant happiness. Go for peace. Weight control really is a possibility when you accept lifelong maintenance as the tool that will bring you to this peace of mind.

Letting Go

You can let go of all your old myths and false hopes by identifying in your questionnaire what your biggest areas of concern are, by actively choosing to forgo them, and then by reminding yourself several times a day that you did it.

Write down the myths that scored a two or three on your quiz and any other personal myths you have identified along the way on separate note cards. Carry these cards around with you. Review them at least three times a day and before you go to bed. Think about your myths and how they are affecting you physically and emotionally. Say to yourself silently or out loud, "I must let go of the myth that—"

Why should you do this? Because your personal myths are habits in thinking, and like all habits, they die hard. You have to work at breaking them at first so that eventually they won't mean anything to you anymore. They'll be like old clothes that you used to wear at another weight.

Do the work now. It will pay off handsomely in the end.

The Hard Truth

Sure, you still have to think about weight control. Although you will never be a chronic dieter again, you will be taking charge of your eating and feelings about your body image. To master this new responsibility, to succeed at maintaining a weight that's right for you, and also to like yourself (something you've probably never done), you will accept the following truths:

- I will never have a perfect body.
- I accept that my weight problem is a chronic condition that will require lifetime attention to control.
- I accept that without attention, my weight problem will automatically reemerge.
- I accept that there is not now and never will be a quick fix or magic solution to my weight problem.
- I accept that food is a necessity and a pleasure and that just by eating small amounts of restricted items I will not necessarily damn myself to obesity forever.
- I accept the fact that the key to my self-esteem is not now and never will be the shape of my body.

Letting go is a conscious decision that results in active behavior. It means that you will not let old beliefs about food work on you, leaving you a passive observer in the great game of life.

You must constantly reinforce the process of letting go of these damaging myths and ideas, particularly because the counterbalance of media hype is everywhere. So what if you keep hearing the message that your sense of worth lies in the way you look? Let go.

So what if the grinning models wearing the new fall fashions tell you that you must be anorexic and emaciated in order to succeed? Let go.

Understand that you've been brainwashed about your body

and what it means in the bigger picture of your life. Just let go.

You will be healthy, feel good physically, and protect yourself from cancer, diabetes, heart disease, osteoporosis, and a host of other ailments by allowing the stress in your life to dissolve as you craft for yourself a new, balanced way to eat and exercise. Let go of the concept that weight loss leads to happiness. That false belief is what keeps you from liking yourself right here, right now, and in succeeding where success counts—in gaining peace of mind.

Knowledge on the Road to Recovery

Now you know. There are biological, mental, psychological, historical, and societal factors at play in the way you look and the way you conduct your eating and exercising behaviors.

Look seriously at the way you react to this knowledge and if you can, at this early stage in the program, try to separate out the real information from your feelings about your own success or failure and your like or dislike of your body.

These are the facts. Use them well and wisely and you will see that on the road to curing your obsession with your weight forever, the truth will serve you well. When you accept what really exists and turn your back on myths, you can effectively change your attitude about Fat Madness.

I Recognize That I Must Approach Weight Loss in a Rational Way

Imagine that you are a good, amateur pianist, about to play a concerto with a local symphony orchestra. You have been out of circulation for a while, having a baby, or maybe running a small business. But having had the itch to perform again, you've been practicing like crazy, and now's the time to see if it paid off.

You are nervous, but you are prepared. As you stand backstage, listening to the orchestra tune up, you briefly review all the things you did in order to get ready for this momentous occasion.

1. You cut your nails.
2. You went back to playing scales, arpeggios, and exercises— with a metronome and without—every day, twice a day.
3. You looked over your repertoire and decided not to try something new and different. You selected a piece you'd performed before and would feel comfortable with.
4. You listened to several great artists' interpretations of this piece.
5. You bought a new dress, one that had plenty of arm and back room, one that let you breathe, and one in which you looked totally devastating.
6. You talked to the conductor for hours about the interpretation of the music and compared notes about the other versions you'd both heard. You kept some of your old ideas and added some of her new ones.

7. You practiced the concerto in segments, breaking it down, doing the transitions. Then you put the first half together. When you felt pretty good about that, you started on the second half.
8. You rehearsed with the orchestra. You got to know at least the first-chair musicians' names by heart. You tape-recorded the orchestra's portion of the piece so you could practice at home.
9. You did stress reduction exercises every day, twice a day.
10. You called everyone you knew (even your old piano teacher) and invited them to the concert.
11. You gave yourself permission not to be perfect on the night of the concert. After all, this would be your first time back.

As you stood there backstage and watched the conductor take her place at the podium, you realized that preparation was everything. Because you had done so much before the actual event, you were ready.

Okay. Change of scene. You are no longer in the concert hall. You are in your bedroom, at the beginning of a new day, thinking about how you're handling Fat Madness. You realize you have some weight to get rid of, but you don't want to do it in the same crazy way you've always done it. Well, you can get ready, just the way you could for a concert performance. The same principles apply.

You cannot launch yourself into the void when you're about to do anything really difficult—whether it's playing the piano in front of hundreds of people, or running a marathon, or getting married, or buying a house, or losing weight. You must be completely prepared so that nothing floors you. You can handle family indifference to your new recovery program, your child's turtle dying, a big Italian wedding, and any number of other glitches without flinching. Preparation makes you strong, as you shall see.

Get Ready

You are now going to prepare to shed some pounds, *if you really need to*. To discover whether you are medically overweight or just have an image of yourself as overweight, I want you to use a new, radical method in order to make your choice. No cheating. If you don't need to lose weight, I want you to strongly consider not losing. Believe me, you'll have a lot of work to do that has nothing at all to do with dieting.

If you choose not to try to lose weight, you may skip Step 5 and flip to Step 6 to begin to work on the maintenance skills of your Fat Madness Recovery Program. The truth of the matter is that if your natural weight (setpoint) is lower than your current weight, you'll lose weight and get into better shape just by changing your eating habits and exercising. I'll show you exactly how to do this in Step 6.

I am assuming that you bought this book because you consider yourself overweight. You are probably a chronic diet book buyer as well as a chronic dieter, so you must have figured that there would be some good dieting advice in here.

You're right. Although I intend to cure you of your addiction to Fat Madness, in addition, I do wish you to be a healthy weight when that happens. This is not a book about being fat and happy and screaming at the rest of the mean, cruel world for being so unreasonable about what they consider to be a gorgeous figure.

Although I completely agree that the brainwashing that goes on in our culture is unfair and prejudicial, you still do want to look and feel your best. I stress *feel*. Your best weight is a weight that makes you feel good physically, regardless of any concerns about how the world sees you. (I hope you're still working on letting go of those myths from Step 3.) If you actually have to lose weight for health reasons and do so, and you maintain that healthy weight, you have every right to feel proud of yourself. This self-confidence and determination will carry over into every other part of your life.

If you don't *need* to lose any weight, but have been walking around for years feeling miserable about the way you look, getting into the Fat Madness Recovery Program will give you the same lift. You see, whatever your reason for reading this book, you will benefit. This is emphatically a one-size-fits-all plan.

If it is medically advisable or if you choose to relieve yourself of some fat tissue, you must be prepared—mentally and physically—to get rid of the pounds that you need to lose (as opposed to pounds you feel compelled to lose) in a sound and rational manner. This is a serious commitment and will take a great deal of hard work, so you have to do it right.

You are not going to starve yourself or create strange alchemical combinations that will miraculously make you thinner overnight. You are not going to skip meals or eat only celery. This is your life. You are dealing with matters that affect your health and the *quality* of your life from here on.

Debulking

Sometimes, if we change the words, we can change our perception about the thought behind the words. Instead of heavily loaded phrases like *weight loss, shedding unwanted pounds,* and the real killer, *dieting,* I'd like you to consider *debulking.*

A sweater is bulky. If you take it off, you have debulked. If you can imagine the excess fat on your body as a heavy winter coat, one that you can shed by the simple physical motions of unbuttoning and rotating your arms and pulling, maybe you'll begin to see the issue from another perspective.

When we talk about debulking, it's not emotional, it's not guilt-producing, and it's not the central challenge of your life. It's not some central life goal that must be accomplished before anything else good can happen. It's just some necessary work that you need to do.

How to Decide If You Need to Debulk

Are you actually medically overweight? Do you really need to debulk? You must first separate out your concerns about health and your concerns about beauty. I am going to show you four ways to do that.

1. Medical reasons. Have you been diagnosed with any of the following conditions?

- Heart disease (or a strong family history of heart disease)
- High serum cholesterol levels (over 200)
- High blood pressure
- Diabetes
- Gallbladder disease
- Arthritis of the weight-bearing joints

If you suffer from any of these conditions, you should consult your physician to set an appropriate weight goal. Overweight people with these diseases do need to lose fat tissue to improve their health, and debulking is like taking a medication that has no side effects.

Reducing fat stores will help to normalize your blood sugar and blood fat levels and control your blood pressure. Debulking can be so successful in doing this that you may not need any other medication. Weight loss also aids and abets a good exercise program, which will get you back into better cardiovascular shape. Medical clearance is absolutely essential if you are suffering from any chronic disease, and I'll deal with that later in this chapter.

2. Measurement technique. If you do not suffer from a chronic disease and are not medically at risk, how else can you judge a potentially dangerous weight situation? You can find out by taking two simple measurements.

The waist-to-hip ratio is crucial in determining where you deposit fat. The areas of fat deposition determine how much of a risk you run by being overweight. As you learned in Step 2, fat above the waist is much more threatening to your health than fat below the waist. Measure your waist and hips. Divide your hip measurement into your waist measurement. For a man, the result should be less than 1; for woman, it should be less than 0.8.

3. *Clothing technique.* What you wear may determine whether you should or shouldn't lose weight. If you purchase your clothes in a regular as opposed to a large-size clothing store, you're on target. That means that if you're a woman and wear anything under a size 18, or if you're a man and wear a suit under a size 48, you're probably fine, and will benefit further from a proper eating and exercise regime. You don't need to debulk.

4. *The new weight table.* Take a look at the weight table on page 95. This is an unusual but absolutely acceptable set of weight ranges based on age and height. If you look at these ranges and think they sound fat to you, *that's madness.* This kind of thinking is not a danger to your physical health, but it certainly is a threat to your mental health.

If you are within or close to range and have not been diagnosed with a disease that can be exacerbated by being overweight, then your only consideration every single time you've dieted has been aesthetics. Remember, you won't radically reshape your body by losing weight.

So, you're fine if you:

1. Don't have a medical problem that might be exacerbated by obesity
2. Have a satisfactory waist-to-hip ratio
3. Wear regular-size clothing
4. Fall near the weight range from the table on page 95. If you are in good health and are not abnormally obese, you may be out of shape, you may have problems with exercising and

maintaining good eating habits, but you are not dangerously fat.

If you are in good health but don't look like your teenage babysitter or the hottest new rock singer, *stop!* Pay attention to the part of your beauty concerns that center around Fat Madness.

Setting Goals—What's Reasonable for You?

Being just a little overweight is not bad for you, and may sometimes be good for you. After fifty, it is healthier to carry five extra pounds as protection around your bones, which become more porous and fragile. At any age, being way below normal weight can be just as dangerous to your health as being way above. Chronic stress causes death, too, and we all know how stressful it is to be constantly preoccupied with dieting and weight. Keep in mind that crossing the street at the wrong time can kill you quicker than any weight problem. I'm not being facetious. I am pointing out that you must have reasonable wishes for your body and goals for your weight range. I will give you ranges that are pretty generous.

What should you weigh? This is really a loaded question. You can see by taking a stroll in any mall that by our society's current standards, 130 pounds might appear to be chunky for a 5'4" woman over fifty, but it looks positively ethereal on a willowy high school basketball star (or emaciated model) standing 5'11". Look at the new weight table on page 95. You can be 5'4" and 130 and you aren't fat. This is a reasonable weight based on a bell-shaped curve that shows fatness and thinness.

What do you mean by fat, anyway? If you look at the chart on page 92, you'll see that for all people, body weights are distributed in the following bell-shaped pattern.

Most people of average weight cluster toward the middle, with the obese and anorexic people hovering on the edges. When you start out with your weight loss goals, see how you adjust this bell-shaped curve to reflect your opinions about what constitutes fat. Helped along by society's values, you forget about the average range and lump everyone who isn't grossly underweight into the fat category. If you're not very thin (too thin, according to the table below), you are fat. What happened to in between?

Go to any mall and take an informal body poll. Try to be scientific; be completely objective and rational. You will notice that people truly do come in all shapes and sizes. The so-called beautiful people are clearly in the vast minority, squeezed into a small corner at the lower end of the bell-shaped curve. And there is a very good chance that a high percentage of the women you see whose bodies do conform to today's standards of beauty are maintaining that shape through anorexic and bulimic behaviors. They want to get to their goal at any cost to their health, whereas you know now that the *real* goal is to get healthy in your mind about how you feel in your body.

The problem with goal setting is that weight is not always the criterion. Someone like Melanie, whom we met back at Step 2, is thin above the waist and rounded below. Were she to diet until she had her bottom looking the way she wanted it, she would have depleted most of her body's necessary fat stores and

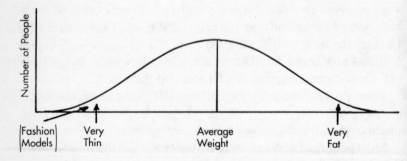

Bell-Shaped Curve Distribution of Body Weights

be dangerously close to starvation.

You cannot always appear the way you wish to appear. You can't look like Michelle Pfeiffer no matter how hard you try. Nor can you fly, invent a cure for cancer by tomorrow, or in most cases, get along with your in-laws. These are things we must live with. By the end of this book, when the entire recovery program comes into full focus, you will be able to accept living with and caring for yourself just as you are.

You are now at the point where you can make some concrete decisions.

1. You can choose your weight range.
2. You will let go of unrealistic weight loss goals (see Step 3 if you need a review). It is unrealistic to select a goal that matches what you weighed in high school or college, or that takes you down to a size you haven't worn in years.
3. You will pick a goal that is reasonable for you. You have the option of selecting no goal, and just figuring out how you've debulked by watching the change in the way your clothing fits.
4. You will gauge yourself not just on what you'd like to look like, but will take life events into account. If you have just been pregnant or you have just passed menopause, your goals must reflect those experiences that cause a natural increase in weight.
5. You will not set an external event as a goal. You are not permitted to diet in order to fit into a bikini by June if it's currently April and you have thirty pounds to go. There are serious medical consequences to this type of dieting, not the least of which is malnutrition.
6. You will remain flexible in your goal setting. If you've been too strict, just as you have been on previous diets in your life, you're going to lighten up. This recovery program will ultimately result in giving you an inner calm and understanding that will help you accept and be proud of whatever you accomplish, even if it is less than you originally hoped for.

How Fast Should You Lose Weight?

All experts say that one of the most crucial factors in weight loss and particularly in maintenance is the rate at which most people shed their pounds. The faster you lose, the more likely you are to put weight back on, and the riskier it is for the rest of your body's systems and organs. Remember that dieting is an unnatural state. You are depriving your body of calories that it thinks it needs, so it goes into overdrive to compensate for being starved. Serious complications of quick weight loss include gall-bladder disease, kidney stones, and depleting the body's organs and muscles of necessary protein.

The best precaution against any medical complications is to *lose slowly on a balanced diet*. One-half to one pound a week is optimal, and you should lose no more than two pounds per week. The first week on any diet, you lose a lot of water, so five pounds is permissible at the very start of your diet, but not after that.

The New Height/Weight Chart

Forget the Metropolitan Life Insurance Company's chart. They have made millions of us miserable with their dictate that all people of all ages should weigh about the same based on some amorphous concept of small, medium, and large frames. These old tables were statistically inaccurate, because in the study on which they based their data, they were measuring only those individuals who bought life insurance, mostly those who worked in white-collar jobs for big companies. This left out at least half the population, the blue- and pink-collar component and all kinds of people who worked for themselves, such as housewives and artists.

You have been living with the wrong ranges that have convinced you that you're heavier for your size than you should be. They only take weight and height into consideration, although you know by now that what really matters is what percentage of your body is fat and where it's located and whether you have any weight-related medical problems.

Try this chart from the National Research Council (1989). I don't want you to think about the numbers in the table as your goal. The table is just an aid, to show you where you sit in the bell-shaped curve.

As you now know, people tend to get a little heavier as they age, and they can safely weigh several more pounds than they carried in high school. The higher weights in the ranges usually apply to men, because they have more muscle and bone.

Suggested Weights For Adults

Height	Weight in Pounds	
	19 to 34 years	*35 years and over*
5'0"	97–128	108–138
5'1"	101–132	111–143
5'2"	104–137	115–148
5'3"	107–141	119–152
5'4"	111–146	122–157
5'5"	114–150	126–162
5'6"	118–155	130–167
5'7"	121–160	134–172
5'8"	125–164	138–178
5'9"	129–169	142–183
5'10"	132–174	146–188
5'11"	136–179	151–194
6'0"	140–184	155–199
6'1"	144–189	159–205
6'2"	148–195	164–210
6'3"	152–200	168–216
6'4"	156–205	173–222
6'5"	160–211	177–228
6'6"	164–216	182–234

Medical Clearance

You should be really healthy before you begin any diet and exercise program. Remember that debulking is an unnatural experience for the body. Depriving yourself of nutrients for the express purpose of losing fat tissue just doesn't make metabolic sense to your organs. Of course, doing nothing but sitting around and eating is also unnatural, but consciously attempting to take away part of yourself isn't what nature intended, either.

Consider the following questions:

1. Are you receiving regular medical care for an ongoing illness?
2. Are you currently taking any prescription medications?
3. Do you have one or more of the following medical conditions?
   Heart disease
   Abnormal heart rhythm
   Diabetes
   High blood pressure
   Gallbladder disease
   Kidney disease
   Arthritis or gout
   Gastrointestinal problems
   Liver disease
   Thyroid or other endocrine disease

If you answered yes to any of these questions, you *must* consult a physician before beginning any weight loss program.

You should also see a physician if:

1. You are considering pregnancy any time in the near future or you are currently nursing a baby. You could seriously

jeopardize your own health or that of your child if you were to go on a diet.

2. You have ever suffered from anorexia nervosa or bulimia. If you think you might have a problem, you probably do. Don't risk another medically unsupervised weight loss.

3. You have a history of medical complications connected to losing weight. If you ever had unusual symptoms associated with a diet you were on in the past, be sure you see a doctor now, to rule out any future ones.

4. You are under eighteen years of age. Children and adolescents should not diet. They are still growing and need more nutrients than adults. A doctor can, however, supervise a good healthy nutrition and exercise plan that will result in debulking.

Even if you don't fit into one of the above categories but still have concerns about starting a diet, you might consider phoning your physician to discuss your proposed weight loss plan with him or her.

This is likewise true for an exercise program, particularly for those couch potatoes who don't even own a pair of walking shoes at the moment. I'll tell you more about medical clearance for exercise in Steps 5 and 6.

Self-Monitoring Skills

Your physician or your scale can be your guides as to how you're doing from week to week, but they cannot help you in the middle of the night when you wake with agonizing cravings and go binge on a whole bag of potato chips, or early in the morning when, instead of jumping up at 6:30 for a brisk walk, you put on the snooze alarm to get twenty more minutes under the covers.

Who is the one to take care of the nitty-gritty, moment-to-moment skills involved in debulking? Who will tell you when you're hungry or satisfied? And who is going to know if your eating has gone out of control and you are losing your focus on your goal? Just you. Only you.

You can do it, as long as you are aware of what you are doing and are able to monitor and track your eating and exercise behaviors accurately. This doesn't always come naturally. As a chronic dieter, you may have lost touch with your monitoring ability. Before you begin debulking, you need to get that back. Otherwise, you may sabotage your own efforts and not even know it. So let's discuss the two basics: *hunger* (when to eat) and *satiety* (when to stop).

Eat When You're Hungry; Stop When You're Comfortably Satisfied

There is a wonderful concept that's been around forever but that seems to have been lost in the miasma of diet-speak. That concept is *satiety*. Being satiated, as opposed to full or stuffed, is a healthy feeling. It means that you've fulfilled yourself, taken care of yourself, and that you have reached a comfort level where you are perfectly content. It's the endpoint of appropriate eating—it feels good and also makes you feel good about yourself. It is the brain's signal to the rest of you announcing that you have vanquished hunger, *not* that you have stuffed your stomach. That is a different signal altogether.

The body registers the presence of food with two separate mechanisms. The first is one that we are all too familiar with, the stretching of the stomach. There's a set of special nerves located in the stomach wall that respond when the walls of the stomach are stretched. They don't care whether you've loaded in five Twinkies or a huge portion of pasta. They don't care about nutrition or great tastes. They just loosen the old belt (so to speak) and make room for a little more. And their response is immediate. They report the presence of food to the brain as soon as it arrives.

The second mechanism for registering the presence of food in the body is the satiety center buried deep in the brain. This specialized group of cells interprets signals delivered from the digestive system to the bloodstream. These signals include nutrients from food and digestive enzymes from the intestines. It takes time for this important information to get through, because the food needs to be in the process of breaking down into its various nutrients for the signal to start up to the brain. This takes about fifteen to twenty minutes.

The sensation that normally stimulates eating is hunger. In fact, you could view eating as a behavior intended to remove the presence of that noxious and uncomfortable feeling.

Now, here's where it gets really interesting. Only the satiety center removes hunger. The stretch receptors in the stomach simply bypass it.

Think about this: You are starving and you wolf down a couple of platefuls of food. What stops you from eating even more? You're now in pain! Your overstretched stomach feels awful. This experience has nothing to do with the absence of hunger. You feel full, not satiated. But fullness is the feeling most chronic dieters use to stop themselves from eating more.

What does pure satiety feel like? Don't tell me you don't know. You've eaten on a plane where you only get so much food and no more. You've eaten in a restaurant that serves reasonable portions.

When you go to eat at a restaurant, you are usually pretty hungry, having saved your appetite for a nice meal. So you order an appetizer, salad, entrée, and dessert. The rolls arrive. You are so hungry that you could eat the whole basket. You don't; you've developed enough discipline to limit yourself to two rolls while waiting for the appetizer. After a seemingly endless wait, the appetizer arrives. It's a small portion of something rich, like pâté or clams oreganata, and you eat it slowly, savoring the taste and texture of the food. You're feeling pretty good now.

Soon the appetizer is replaced by the salad, which you also enjoy, along with another roll. You begin to notice that you aren't ravenous anymore. You're not stuffed; you wouldn't even call yourself full, but you are not hungry. This, of course, is a dilemma because when the expensive entrée arrives, you don't really feel like eating it.

You have now arrived at the state of satiety, the absence of hunger. You feel comfortable with the amount of food you had because the restaurant paced your eating for you and gave your brain a chance to tell you that you were satiated before you had a chance to overstretch your stomach. Notice that you have satisfied your hunger with a lot less food than you might have eaten at home. (Of course, most of us go on to down that entrée and lose the feeling of satiety as we stuff ourselves once again.)

If you eat to satiety and then stop eating, you will never gain a pound. Since you probably rarely stopped at your point of satiation, but went on eating until you were over-full, *with this new procedure, you will lose weight.* Your body processes get a break because they're not tied up with digesting excess amounts of food.

Here are some of the benefits of eating just enough: Your insulin levels will be stable, your blood glucose will not fluctuate markedly, and all the cells of your body will get their ration of glucose and nutrients at a nice steady level. Your glycogen stores will level out and be ready to deliver their burst of energy when needed by the muscles. Your kidneys and liver will be saved the burden of overwork. They won't be prematurely damaged by having to digest, metabolize, and excrete the great amounts of toxins that come along with great amounts of excess food, and they will be able to keep up with the many processes they must perform.

As the mechanics of your body work better, you will be better able to respond to the signals that evolution built into your brain: *Ah,* the brain admits. *I thought I was hungry and I was. I ate to relieve that hunger and now, I'm satiated.* Basta. *Enough.*

You will find that knowing your satiation level gives you a powerful tool against compulsive, binge, or secret eating. Evidently, if you have to think consciously about what you're doing to satisfy your hunger, you can't eat blindly. And when you are

eating with the goal of making yourself feel better physically—
when you're thinking as opposed to just doing—you enhance
rather than depress your self-confidence.

As you get into the swing of knowing when you've hit that
level, you further contribute to your own well-being.

Experiment right now, assuming you haven't just stuffed
yourself and you are at least moderately hungry. I want you to
eat one piece of fruit, slowly. One lovely complex carbohydrate
with good taste—apple, banana, pear, peach, bunch of grapes—
you call the shots.

Wait twenty minutes and do a self-check. You will find that
your hunger is gone or at least greatly reduced, your stomach
isn't stretched or full, you aren't tired or drowsy, but in fact are
probably more alert and energized and *not thinking about food*.
Welcome to the world of satiety. (Hint: Try eating the piece of
fruit just before you go to the supermarket. You'll see how much
more sensibly you shop.)

Satiety is a barometer of the way in which you feed yourself.
You have to be conscious to realize when you're satiated. You
can't just sit blankly in front of a TV and put things in your
mouth and chew and swallow. You have to think. This is also
important in conjunction with exercise, which we get to in Step
6. Evidently, if you're stuffed, it's impossible for you to get up
from the table and go take a brisk walk. So if you feed your
body wrong, you can't achieve the state of fitness you want to
be in.

Try satiety again. This time, wait until lunch. Prepare a nice
sandwich—maybe turkey or tuna or cheese on whole-grain
bread, possibly spread with mustard. You might want a salad to
go with it. Cut the sandwich in half, and put one half in the
refrigerator. Consciously sit down, and eat what's in front of
you. Take a walk around the block, or make a phone call.

Return to your dining room or office desk. How do you feel?
Are you still hungry? Do you have gnawing hunger pangs, or
are you just feeling like a nibble? If so, take the second half of
your sandwich out and cut that in half. Put the last quarter in

the refrigerator and eat the quarter that's in front of you. (This is the half-life theory of sandwich consumption.)

At this point, I bet you're satiated. And the only way you can tell is to do this exercise faithfully on a regular basis, really examining the way you feel after you've put food in your mouth, chewed it, swallowed it, and waited for your brain, not your stomach, to tell you if you've had enough.

Your Hunger/Satiety Diary

Many diet gurus counsel you to keep a diary of everything you eat, where you eat it, the time, the amount, and the emotion you're feeling. To my way of thinking, this places undue emphasis on the act of eating, which should be a pleasurable experience. Besides, who wants to fill out reams of multicolumned worksheets every day? What a waste of valuable time and energy!

I believe in keeping things simple. And I do believe that a hunger/satiety diary is a great idea. It's a reminder that you're awake and aware. If you have a daily reminder book or weekly schedule minder, you can get it to perform a double duty.

After you've eaten or, if you prefer, at the end of the day, write down what you ate. Don't bother with the exact serving size or calorie count, just record what you ate during each eating period in very general terms. Then rate your hunger before you ate and your feeling of satisfaction afterward. Do it on the following scale:

	Hunger Scale	**Satiety Scale**
One:	STARVING	STILL HUNGRY
Two:	MODERATELY HUNGRY	COMFORTABLY SATISFIED
Three:	NOT HUNGRY	FULL OR STUFFED

Sample Hunger/Satiety Diary

Food	Hunger Number	Satiety Number
Breakfast: Orange juice, blueberry muffin, coffee	2	2
Snack: Potato chips	3	3
Lunch: Egg salad sandwich, Coke, donut	1	3
Dinner: Pork chops, mashed potatoes, beans, ice cream	1	3
Snack: Leftover chili, crackers	3	2
Snack: Peanut butter sandwich, Oreos, milk	2	3

You may find that despite its simplicity, this diary isn't easy to fill in. It may be difficult for you to rank your hunger because you may have lost your awareness of subtle differences in hunger after years of chronic dieting. This is to be expected.

It also might not be easy to face what you are eating each day when it is written down in black and white. That's normal, too. Most chronic dieters develop patterns of denial. They ignore or choose not to remember exactly what and how much they are eating. Don't despair. In time you'll learn to be conscious of your food consumption. Be patient with yourself.

Giving Yourself Time to Catch Up

The drug addict and alcoholic stop growing emotionally the day they start abusing drugs. Their recovery must include some catching up, where they discover their emotional maturity levels and slowly, painfully climb this ladder back to sanity and sobriety. Grown-ups have to relearn some very elementary social skills; teens have to get out of the bad patterns of arrested development that have kept them in the vicious cycle of abuse.

Chronic dieters face similar challenges. Remember that if you've been beating yourself over the head for years about food and what you look like, you've lost the ability to judge rationally what and how much is appropriate to eat. Now you're going to have to relearn how to feel hunger and eat in response to that; and then you're going to have to learn how to stop eating when you're comfortably satisfied with what you've consumed.

Your diary is the first step. Keep it going for at least a week. It will teach you about your food choices, about the way you eat, and about what it is that triggers you to start and stop eating. Learning all this will not happen overnight. It requires a great deal of attention.

It's particularly hard to relearn hunger. When you're actually consuming food based on your hunger as opposed to your cravings or boredom or any of the many other stimuli that get your mouth moving mindlessly, you can get frustrated and confused. If you decide to debulk, you're going to be in a state of caloric deprivation, so you'll have to deal with hunger every day. This is not fun, but it will also give you an opportunity to relearn the ways in which you experience hunger and how you can use it as a guide to determine when you should eat. Your eventual goal is to keep your hunger and satiety level at a 2 on the above scale as much as possible.

These are big changes, but you'll make them. Remember that recovery is a lifelong process and the less you push for it, the more easily it will come to you.

Time to Choose

At the beginning of this step, I asked you to think about whether you choose to debulk. You were asked to decide whether to shed pounds on a formal diet program or to simply move on to healthier eating and exercise behaviors as your lifetime plan for weight control.

Have you made your choice? Are you comfortable with it? If you've had it with diets and don't need to debulk for any of the reasons we specified at the beginning of this chapter, skip to Step 6 to learn how to develop comfortable and maintainable changes in your eating and exercise habits. If you are sure you want to debulk, it's time to move on to Step 5.

Still not sure? That's okay. You have the power to make a choice whenever you want and to change your mind even after you choose. You don't need diet experts to coerce you into doing something that's not right for you. How does it feel to be treated with respect, to treat yourself with respect? Pretty good, I'll bet. A lot better than causing yourself needless agony about how you look, how you behave, and what others think about you.

Remember, your worst problem isn't your weight, it's your self-esteem. Every step in your Fat Madness Recovery Program is designed to prioritize the goal of recapturing your feelings of self-worth and personal effectiveness. This choice is part of that process.

Your diet—the way that you actually accomplish the debulking—is *not* a priority. Lifetime maintenance of a serene and self-confident attitude is.

Now you are prepared to debulk if you need to. You've got your tools, your mindset, and all the time in the world. Your next step is to select the right plan.

■ STEP 5: DEBULK

I Know That Losing Pounds Is Only the Beginning

You are now more than halfway through the Fat Madness Recovery Program and you have done the necessary hard work that will help you in this most difficult step. You now fully understand the nature of your weight control problem and have worked through your denial. You have a nuts-and-bolts working knowledge of the facts about nutrition and have sorted out the psychological mishmash about food and body image that came down to you from your family, the media, and society. You are in the process of letting go of the myths and false hopes that have sabotaged your ability to control your weight up to this point. You've set yourself a realistic goal and you're truly prepared to achieve it.

Congratulations! Now comes the lousy part.

THE CHOICE TO DEBULK IS YOURS AND NO ONE ELSE'S

If you have to for medical reasons or feel that you wish to, you are going to debulk.

Understand that this is your choice. No one in the world can tell you that you have to lose weight or that you owe it to yourself to make another valiant attempt to alter your body. I am telling you that debulking can *assist* you in getting rid of your

Fat Madness, but it is only one step—the least important and the most uncomfortable step—in nine.

It is by no means the linchpin of this program. It is merely a spoke in the wheel, and it won't be missed if you remove it. The wheel will turn anyhow. If you find that it is too painful to go through the deprivation and hardship of limiting what you eat one more time, then you have the option of not doing so. It's up to you.

Debulking is an unnatural behavior for the body. Your metabolic processes are thrown for a loop every time you deny them their proper caloric input. Your whole system screams for help. The body doesn't understand why you are radically altering the amount of nutrients you put into it. Maybe you're trying to starve it to death. Maybe it should just shut down to conserve everything it's got. Maybe it should hungrily remind you on a very regular basis just how lousy it feels without the amounts of food it's used to.

Losing weight is tough, as it should be. If it wasn't so hard, people would forget to eat and become malnourished and fade away. If we didn't have that chronic sensation of hunger, we wouldn't take care of the body's business, which is to maintain equilibrium and repair and replenish cells for growth and health.

So let's be real. Debulking is a painful experience, causing hunger pangs, weakness, fatigue, headache, crankiness, and depression (and I'll bet you can you think of even more symptoms you've experienced on numerous diets). The desire to avoid these symptoms helps to explain why so many dieters gain back so much weight before they're willing to face that pain again. Then how do you do it? Is there any secret to debulking?

The secret is to be aware of your own particular nutsiness around this issue. If you do choose to debulk, you should do so in any reasonable, rational, healthful fashion that works for you, not something that's worked for your best friend, aunt, or mother-in-law, and certainly not something that's touted to the skies on television. You know yourself, and you know the little slips and dodges you make when you diet. So pick the system that is most comfortable for you and that causes you the least amount of pain. This may be a method that's worked for you in the past, or it may be something entirely new. In most cases, you should lose slowly and gradually. If it takes months, it takes months; it's not a race. Debulking is a step that you will accomplish and then put behind you. You will only be doing it this one, final time.

THE PHYSICAL SIDE OF DEBULKING: HOW THE BODY LOSES WEIGHT

Let's take apart the weight loss process so you'll be able to make an informed decision about how you'd like to facilitate this process. You are in charge. You're the captain of this ship, and you get to steer it the way you want to, on a true course toward change.

You know the following information, but I'll repeat it so that you can see what debulking is actually doing to your poor maligned metabolism. If you consume fewer calories than you expend, you lose weight. And how do you lose it?

All About Weight, or What Makes You Heavy?

Everything you are weighs something: your heart, your lungs, your muscles, your fat, your bones, and particularly, your water content. Water's terribly heavy. If you're drinking a healthy six to eight glasses a day, you may know this already from lifting those six-gallon bottles onto your water cooler. Your body is 70 percent water, and that represents a lot of your poundage.

When you stand on the scale after the first week of debulking, you often see a radical decrease, perhaps as much as five or eight pounds. The scale doesn't know what part of your body you've lost, and it doesn't care. You lose your water first, then fat, then, in extreme and unhealthy dieting situations, you lose protein. Losing protein is bad since it means losing tissue from all your vital organs, like the heart. Loss of essential body tissue can seriously compromise your health and well-being.

Let's get back to the beginning of your debulking process and talk a little about water weight. All these gallons of water in your body are stored in two compartments, but the water can move freely between these two areas. There is *intracellular* water, right inside the cells, where most of it is stored, and *extra-cellular* water. When you deprive your body of carbohydrates, as you do on a diet, the intracellular water shifts to the extra-cellular spaces, and this dilutes the blood. When this occurs, your body is in a state of *diuresis*.

The kidneys, which remove excess fluids and the toxins contained within them from the body, become aware of this imbalanced state and begin working hard to equalize the cells and get the blood back to its normal consistency. They pump that extra-cellular water right out the bladder. You know how often you have to urinate on the first week of your diet and how almost clear and colorless the urine can be. This is because it's in an extremely dilute state.

So there you are, losing water right and left. You shed pounds immediately, and you actually feel thinner—even your clothes fit better. This is because subcutaneous water and water contained in your fat tissue typically give you that bloated feeling, especially during your period. Now—at least temporarily—it's gone. Of course the upsetting part of all this is that you haven't lost much fat yet, and the pounds that have poured off into the toilet are easily regained if you should happen to reintroduce carbohydrates—which cause you to retain water—to your diet. You may have lost five to eight pounds your first week, but these will pop right back on if you deviate at all from your restricted eating.

How do you get around this problem? Always drink six to eight glasses of water a day while you're debulking *and* afterward, to maintain the appropriate water balance in your body. You won't lose as much in your first week, but you won't have that false sense of water loss being real loss, either.

Using the Scale

This is a real personal choice, and it's unfortunately a choice that has probably been feeding into your Fat Madness for years. Some people weigh themselves constantly when they're on a diet. Some go and stand on the scale five or even ten times a day. You're compelled to look, the way you're drawn to stare at a car accident on the highway. And you're compelled to revisit the scene of the crash over and over again. Even though the circumstances don't change, and the crunch of metal and tinkle of glass are the same, you want to give it just one more look.

"Did it really say 145 when I woke up this morning? I had an incredibly tiny lunch and I drank all my water, so maybe I'm down to 140." Wishful thinking, plain and simple. The body remains practically constant through several days of processing nutrients and excreting water and toxins.

The scale won't tell you anything helpful if you use it more than once a week. It may depress the heck out of you even if you use it that infrequently. But it is your choice—yours alone—and you may choose to use the scale in whatever manner you wish. Here's what a scale can do.

On the negative side:

1. It can give you a false sense of weight loss.
2. It can (and often does) give you an inaccurate reading.
3. It can be the source of incentive to deal with the deprived feelings during debulking if you lose weight, but it can also cause you to get discouraged and give up if you gain.
4. It can mislead you, since weight loss is not a linear process. There will be days when you don't lose, days when you even gain a little, even in strict debulking. Your body is variable and flexible. A pound lost is not a finished product.
5. The scale may set up expectations in your mind that simply can't be met.

On the positive side:

1. It can act as a barometer of how well you are suited to the weight loss program you've selected.
2. It can give you a weekly ritual (something to do at the same time of day in the same state of undress), that can serve as a numerical reward for your efforts.
3. It can give you an objective measurement to see if you're plateauing or reaching your setpoint.

You know that if you use the scale one or more times a day, any variation you see is just water shifting around. Changes in fat content take much longer. Let's figure this out. There are about 3,500 calories of energy in each pound of fat, which means you'd need to create a deficit of 3,500 calories before a pound of fat could get out of storage and start to deliver fuel to your body.

The United States Department of Agriculture (USDA) guidelines tell us that women need an average of 1,600 calories a day to maintain their weight. Even a teenage boy only consumes 2,800 for the same purpose. Even *he*—jumping around and burning through his raging hormones—can't lose a pound of fat in a day. Since the most perfectly balanced scale gives a reading to within only one pound of accuracy, you can see that daily use makes no sense. It is madness to monitor tiny increments of water shifting around as your incentive to debulk. You need some real, thoughtful incentives (your health, your sanity, the fact that you won't have to do this again once you're in control of your Fat Madness) instead. Who cares what your scale says?

Here's an option. Don't use the scale at all. It's caused you pain, humiliation, and defeat in the past. You'll know from your clothes whether you're losing. Radical, huh? Consider trying it. It might work for you.

What Kind of Diet Is Best for Debulking?

You may use any diet at all that provides a *balance of nutrients*. Most of the commercial diet programs and influential diet books these days give excellent advice on how to mix and match the right amounts of *macronutrients* (carbohydrates, protein, and fat) and *micronutrients* (vitamins and minerals). Different programs will fit you out with different proportions of these, but sound nutritionists advocate that you eat over half of your daily calories in complex carbohydrates; less than 20 percent in protein, preferably vegetable rather than animal protein, since animal protein comes marbled with fats; and from 20 percent to 30 percent in fats.

Micronutrients, which may or may not be supplemented, should include Vitamin A, all the B's, C, D, E, K, folate (folic acid), and niacin. Your minerals should include calcium (particularly for women), phosphorus, magnesium, iron, potassium, selenium, and zinc.

Getting this good balance ensures that your body processes will go on normally, particularly your protein turnover, which is so essential to your metabolic function and to the repair and restoration of the body. The amount of protein broken down should be equal to the amount being built up. If it's not, you're losing tissue from your vital organs and muscles. In extreme cases, such as severe anorexia, this can lead to the body literally eating itself up.

Some fat in your diet is necessary, though nowhere nearly as much as you undoubtedly consume on a regular basis (about 40 percent to 50 percent of the typical American diet is made up of fats). Fats don't just make you fat. They have their purposes as you learned in Step 2 and one of these is helping you to assimilate and absorb vitamins. So some fat is necessary and any sound diet program will include it.

Why Do You Reach Plateaus When You Debulk?

There are as many variations in the rate of weight loss and in the timing of plateaus as there are dieters. Your body is a bio-chemical factory that chugs along at its own pace, and it will not cooperate when you decide to change its natural inclination to keep the metabolism going *its* way. The body stops losing and then loses again for unknown reasons. It can be holding onto water (for example, when you have your period), it can be reaching your setpoint weight so it can't lose any more, or it might be reacting to a decrease in physical activity. If you've been conserving energy to the point where your calories in are equal to your calories out, you're not burning excess fuel, so you stop losing weight.

Pushing through a plateau requires patience. It may also re-quire a new realization of your true setpoint. Maybe you just weren't intended physiologically to be a size 8 or 10. You'll have to accept your real weight possibilities and live with them. Another suggestion to get off your plateau is to get off your buns and really start moving. If you increase your caloric ex-penditure with exercise, you will eventually begin to lose again. (See Step 6 for a careful and reasonable exercise plan.)

The Psychology of Debulking: How It Feels to Deprive Yourself

What a terrible feeling! Deprivation stinks. As many times as you've lost weight, as many times as you've sat yourself down and made that crucial decision to grocery shop like a monk and eat like a bird, it's always agonizing. You know you have to limit your calories and portions, and you have to watch yourself every single moment. You have to make your hunger vanish or deny it or figure out some reward for not giving in to it. When you impose this kind of rigid self-discipline, you begin to rankle.

At any moment, you could pick up that ball and chain that's hung around your refrigerator door and crash right through.

What is this feeling of desperation? Of course, you're hungry. But it's not just a physical hunger, it's also a psychological hunger, a perfectly understandable craving for the foods and quantities you're denying yourself. But there is also Fat Madness lurking here. If you continue to define yourself as being morally good because you didn't eat, or because you didn't eat what you really craved, or because you stopped eating before you devoured Cleveland, that's not quite sane, is it? How will you define yourself when you give in to the craving and cheat?

The psychological side of the deprivation equation is the true source of anguish during debulking. The internal assault on your self-worth hurts much more than any physical hunger ever could. That is why it is important to find a way to comply with a debulking plan as much as possible, and that is why so many diverse diet programs are commercial successes. It has little or nothing to do with the actual nuts and bolts of their debulking plans. They all involve delivering fewer calories to the body than it needs. There are no secrets. The major difference between all diet programs revolves around their particular methods of helping the dieter deal with the psychological issues of deprivation.

Different diet programs have different methods of making it easier for you to cope with deprivation. There's no reason for you to stick with a program that sets your teeth on edge. The diet programs that are successful generally work because of their psychological mechanisms for helping the dieter deal with loss—not weight loss, but loss of comfort. Since everyone's psyche is different, the more you prioritize your particular needs during the debulking process, the more readily you can find the plan that's just right for you.

Mary, one of my patients, told me that she has to have a small taste of something she loves once a day. Just a taste and she can put the rest away. A restrictive program forbidding certain foods is absolutely wrong for Mary. She prefers to eat one piece of pizza for lunch than twenty slices of turkey breast. Mary needs a very liberal program, because she's great at self-monitoring.

Joe, on the other hand, finds that the stimulation of tastes he craves drives him to distraction. If he tried the one-slice method, he'd end up eating the whole pizza and ordering a second to go. For Joe, it's best to have plain, bland foods—even a liquid meal once a day. (Many of the folks who've lost mammoth amounts of weight on physician-directed Optifast or Medifast programs say that they lost their appetite when they were drinking their shakes because they had no psychological stimulation to eat.)

Sally, who has successfully lost weight time and again (and successfully gained it back time and time again), says she needs to feel she's not in a vacuum when she's debulking. She has to have the support of other people who, like herself, are going through the weight loss process. For Sally, the Weight Watchers meeting gives her a forum for sharing with others. She's allowed to have the feeling that she's doing well with her deprivation, and this motivates her to continue.

April is an inveterate cook who loves preparing elaborate feasts for family and friends. Her debulking program has to offer her real foods and a chance to tinker with cooking methods and new low-fat and low-calorie recipes. She thrives on a program that offers creative menus and exchanges of one meal possibility for another—a kind of Chinese banquet approach to deprivation.

There is some program out there that will work well for you. Maybe you've already used it; maybe you haven't yet hit on the one that's going to make debulking as palatable as it can be for you. We're going to recommend a few of the most successful in each category. You can certainly lose in other ways—for example, eating exactly half of everything you eat now (restricting portion as opposed to substance). Or beefing up your exercise program and continuing to eat as you do. This takes longer, but it is a very healthy option that I heartily recommend.

Just remember, as you read on, that if you select a program to help you debulk, you must have a *balanced diet* and a *significant period of time* to lose your weight. It's okay to take more time. You'll never have to do this step again if you do it right now.

THE DIETS

Very Low Calorie vs. Low Calorie

Diets come in two categories: *VLCDs (Very Low Calorie Diets,* which are under 1,000 calories per day) and *LCDs (Low Calories Diets,* which are usually from 1,000 to 1,800 calories a day).

VLCDs are medically supervised modified fasting plans that may deliver as few as 450 calories daily. They are often mistakenly called liquid diets because the calories are usually offered as liquid shakes or drinks that you consume four or five times daily. There is occasionally some solid food involved, but not much, and it's not very tasty. These diets are the outcome of years of research in fasting. Obesity experts saw that you can't simply shut the body down in order to achieve a big drop in pounds; you have to replace some nutrients at the lowest level.

These diets, also known as *protein-sparing modified fasts,* should be used only if you are fifty pounds overweight or need to lose at least 50 percent of your body weight in order to get down to a healthy range. The reason for this is because, as you see, a VLCD is a pretty drastic method of losing, and its safety and effectiveness have been tested only in heavier people. (These diets are not recommended for people with mild or moderate obesity because a greater percentage of the weight they lose is protein. This can be dangerous.)

VLCDs have to be medically supervised because there may be a risk of medical complications. Many factors come into play when a person who may already have a compromised health profile because of obesity loses a great deal of weight via a completely unnatural method of taking in nutrients.

If you are considering this type of diet, you need to find a physician who knows all about VLCDs. Don't consider asking your family doctor unless he has lots of experience with VLCDs or can refer you to somebody who does. You can't just stop a VLCD on your own. You must taper off and learn to eat again since your metabolism has been radically altered and your body isn't used to food anymore.

The following program is an example of a widely available VLCD:

Medifast

This medically supervised program is offered at approximately 8,000 sites nationwide by private physicians and hospitals. Staff always includes a physician and, at the larger centers, a dietician and behavioral consultant as well.

Medical clearance. In your first day of orientation, you'll be examined by the staff doctor who will weigh you. Tests include an EKG, blood and urine analysis, blood pressure reading, and at some sites, a total body fat scan reading.

Weekly weight loss is typically three pounds for women; four to five pounds for men. The protein component of the powdered supplement is about 50 percent for women; 60 percent for men.

Week one to sixteen (in most cases). Women take five packets a day of Medifast 55, with fifty-five grams of protein. The supplement is mixed with six to eight ounces of a noncaloric beverage such as water, club soda, or another sugar-free drink. Men consume the same number of packets of Medifast 70, containing seventy grams of protein. The total caloric intake of the five packets in each category is about 450.

Week sixteen to twenty-two—refeeding. In addition to the packets, all debulkers consume four ounces of lean protein.

Week seventeen. A salad (a cup of raw vegetables) is added.

Week eighteen. Cooked vegetables (½ cup) are added.

Week nineteen. One packet of supplement is eliminated; one fruit is added.

Week twenty. One cup of nonfat milk is added.

Week twenty-one. One bread or cereal is added.

Week twenty-two onward. All powdered supplement is eliminated.

Week twenty-three to thirty-nine—maintenance. A dietician will customize a diet for you.

During all stages of the program, you are counseled one-on-one for medical and emotional support. You meet biweekly with the supervising physician and there is a weekly weigh-in. You may also attend group meetings with a health care provider on staff.

Costs. The initial phases of the diet cost about $65 to $85 a week, depending on location. The Maintenance phase is about $19 a week. The total cost of the forty-week program is about $1,880, which doesn't cover blood tests. Most insurance carriers will reimburse you for office visits and other medical tests.

Other well known VLCDs include Optifast, HMR, and United Weight Control. No research has demonstrated superiority of one program over another. There are also other less well-known VLCD programs. The general principles to keep in mind when considering the VLCD option are:

· They are designed for people with serious weight problems.
· They are expensive.
· They have a high drop-out rate.
· They must be medically supervised by an experienced physician.

LCDs come in all shapes and sizes, just like we do. In this category, we have:

· Prepackaged plans (such as Jenny Craig and Nutri/System)
· Exchange plans, where you select your own foods from lists of choices (such as Deal-a-Meal, Weight Watchers, and the American Dietetic Association diets)

- Meal substitution plans that include one or two liquid meals a day and a suitable solid meal that offers you a balance of calories (such as Slimfast)

THE PROGRAMS

Prepackaged Foods

Nutri/System

This is the most financially successful of all prepackaged debulking plans. There are about 1,800 centers in the United States, Canada, England, and Australia.

Medical clearance. If you're over fourteen and over 10 percent above your ideal body weight or if you have more than seven pounds to lose, if you are not pregnant, and if you are not taking antidepressant medication or diuretics, you may enroll in Nutri/System.

There is no medical exam, but if you suffer from heart disease, kidney disease, diabetes, or have a history of anorexia or bulimia, you need a note from your physician to enroll.

Day 1—orientation. You are asked to fill out questionnaires about food preferences and your health history. A food program is customized for you based on your answers. There are 340 menu variations and 100 foods in the Nutri/System program, and you must purchase all your food from Nutri/System Meal Plans. The foods are approximately 60 percent complex carbohydrate, 20 percent protein, 17 percent fats, and some sodium and fiber.

The plan gives you 1,100 to 1,500 calories a day, including three meals and three snacks. In addition, you can eat unlimited nonstarchy vegetables, two glasses of nonfat milk, two fruits, and a cup of starchy vegetable. You are advised to drink eight glasses of water a day.

Weight loss phase (as long as it takes). You are weighed at your center once a week, and at this time you pick your food choices for the following week. You also have a weekly ten-minute meeting with a diet counselor, who is not a registered dietician, but rather an employee trained in the Nutri/System method. There are weekly thirty-minute Behavior Breakthrough meetings, as well.

Maintenance phase I (as soon as desired amount of weight is lost for eight weeks). You now graduate to eating Nutri/System foods only four times a week, and your own choice of foods the rest of the time. Your diet must encompass your individualized 1,500- to 2,500-calorie-a-day program.

Maintenance phase II (week nine onward). You now eat Nutri/System foods only two days a week, and your own choice the rest of the time.

You may elect a year of supervised maintenance, which includes weekly meetings with a nutritional counselor and a behavioral counselor for the first two months of the year, then biweekly meetings for months three to six, and monthly meetings for months six to twelve.

Costs. The basic weight loss program cost is $89, and for a maintenance program, you will pay an additional $89. (Lifetime enrollment costs about $349.) The foods you must purchase are extra and will cost $57 to $69 a week until you're halfway to your goal weight. Thereafter, as you eat fewer Nutri/System meals, it's about $55 a week. A year-long maintenance program averages approximately $17 a week.

Is Nutri/System for you? You don't have to think about food choices on this program because it's all done for you, so you avoid all food-selection–oriented stimulation. You will do well on this program if it's difficult for you to shop and cook for yourself and not cheat. (Of course, if you're the food preparer for the rest of your family, you'll still have that chore.) You can travel, since you may purchase products at any of the 1,800 locations, but you can't eat in restaurants. The quality and expertise of the staff varies from site to site; and there is no formal exercise program, although debulkers are encouraged to move around. (You are given an aerobics tape in your behavioral training sessions.)

Jenny Craig

This program is offered at 500 centers in the United States, Canada, and Mexico as well as several in Australia (where the program began) and New Zealand.

Medical clearance. If you have at least ten pounds to lose, and do not have multiple food allergies, you may enroll in the program (there are separate programs for children ages eight through seventeen). If you have been diagnosed with heart or kidney disease or diabetes, you must have a doctor's approval to join this program.

The meals supply women with about 1,000 to 1,700 calories daily, and they can lose one to two pounds a week. The meals offer men 1,200 to 1,700 calories, and they can lose two to three pounds a week.

Orientation. At your first meeting with your counselor (a trained employee, not a dietician), you are given a computerized calculation of your weight loss schedule. In this way you know how long it should take you to reach your goal. Caloric levels are adjusted, depending on your needs. Your meal plans are determined at this time. You are also given a multiple vitamin and mineral supplement.

The foods are usually frozen or canned, and there are snacks you can carry with you during the day for a caloric total of 1,000 for women; 1,200 for men. The calories are 60 percent complex carbohydrates, 20 percent protein, 20 percent fat, with some sodium and fiber.

First half of weight loss plan (until you have lost half your desired number of pounds). You eat only Jenny Craig foods and attend a twenty-minute weekly session with your counselor as well as a forty-minute lifestyle class with your peers where you discuss dieting issues and review videotapes about weight loss.

Second half of weight loss. You use Jenny Craig foods

only five days a week and the other days you select your own foods from individualized menu plans that let you make food exchanges among fresh fruit and vegetables, breads, cereals, and low-fat dairy products. By this point, women usually eat their goal weight times thirteen; men usually eat their goal weight times fifteen with a caloric minimum of 1,200 for women; 1,500 for men.

Maintenance (as long as you like). You are weighed monthly and attend a lifestyle class to promote good eating and exercise habits. The discussions have a psychological bent and discuss obsessive eating behavior. A walking program is recommended as an initial physical activity (you can buy a cassette and exercise booklet).

Costs. The company is always running promotional specials, and if you get one, you'll end up paying $1 a pound in program fees. Initially, your sign-up fee is about $70 and you pay an additional $65 to $85 a week for food when you're eating it every day (this cost is halved when you're only eating it half the week).

Is Jenny Craig for you? The advantage of this plan is that you are weaned gradually back onto making your own food choices, so you have the time to learn to think sensibly about shopping and preparation. The counseling sessions stress behavior modification and awareness about food; however, the counselors are not registered dieticians or psychologists. Because you can buy your foods at any center around the country, you can also travel, and you're given guidelines so that you can eat in restaurants during the second half of the program.

Exchange Diets

Weight Watchers

This well-known program claims to be a lifestyle rather than a dieting program: It's dedicated to people with chronic weight control problems. You can buy Weight Watchers meals, snacks, and other foods in any supermarket. The meetings, which offer the kind of support given at Alcoholics Anonymous can be found in many convenient locations, and new groups spring up all the time. There is also an exercise plan and lots of written material to take home.

Medical clearance. You may enroll if you are over ten years old and have at least fifteen pounds to lose. If you have a serious medical condition, you must have your doctor's approval.

Orientation. You set your own weight loss goal based on the Weight Watchers Goal Weight Chart, and then you begin your Personal Choice Program, depending on how much freedom you like in your food planning. On either plan, you will lose about one to two pounds a week. The components of the diet are 50 to 60 percent complex carbohydrates, 20 percent protein, and less than 30 percent fats, with some sodium and fiber.

The *Quick Control Food Plan* dictates the specific foods you will eat, giving you a calorie range of 1,000 to 1,200 for women and 1,400 to 1,500 for men. There are two sets of menus in this plan, and you can switch between them for more variety.

The *Full Choice Plan* is for those who want more control over their food preparation. There are three different levels of caloric intake possible, and you decide which is right for you based on a questionnaire that covers issues like stress level and lifestyle needs. For the first week of your program, you stay at one level; during the second week, you take the questionnaire again and switch levels if you like. At every level, choices are divided into specific portions and include milk, fat, protein, vegetables, fruit, and bread.

On all plans and at all levels, you're advised to eat three meals a day plus snacks and drink six to eight glasses of water.

Maintenance. When you reach your goal weight, you get a maintenance plan booklet, which gives helpful tips on eating, exercising, and problem solving. If you maintain your goal weight for six weeks, you automatically become a lifetime member of Weight Watchers.

Food diaries are recommended, and so are the weekly meetings, which are the cornerstone of the organization. There are weekly community-based meetings, commuter meetings, workplace meetings, and special programs for large groups.

Costs: Your one-time registration fee is from $15 to $18, depending on the site; then you can add $9 to $12 per weekly meeting fee. The foods themselves, available in supermarkets, run from $1.99 on up.

Is Weight Watchers for you? This is a very convenient de-bulking plan. You can buy the foods everywhere, you can use the Weight Watchers cookbook to prepare your own food, and you can attend meetings anywhere in the world. There are certain restaurants that even include Weight Watchers meals on their menus. Exercise is also emphasized here, and there are plans and booklets to teach you how to work out effectively and safely. There are lots of incentives like ribbons and stars along the way as you achieve different goals. If you like group support, this is the organization for you. They will even be there for you in the middle of the night when you're having your worst cravings.

Deal-a-Meal and American Dietetic Association

These food-exchange programs are also ways to learn to control caloric intake by exchanging one item for another of equal caloric value. Deal-a-Meal's popularity is related to the fact that it is promoted by Richard Simmons, whom I greatly admire, by the way, for being the first diet guru to demonstrate any true compassion for the plight of the overweight. The plan simplifies the exchange concept by asking you to deal yourself a certain number of exchange cards per day. When they are gone, you are done eating.

The American Dietetic Association and similar plans are the ones used in most medical offices and by many dieticians and nutritionists. They again involve lists of calorically equivalent exchanges (for instance, one slice of bread is equivalent to half a bagel) to help you plan a low-calorie, balanced diet.

These diets work well for people whose psychological needs during deprivation are best met by complex planning, preparation, and freedom of choice. If these are exactly the opposite of your emotional needs during debulking, these exchange diets will drive you nuts.

Meal Substitutions

Slimfast

There has been some understandable confusion about this liquid meal substitution diet. Because it is liquid, many people have confused it with the VLCD liquid diets. It is not the same. The caloric intake on this meal-substitution plan is at least 1,000 calories a day, making it an LCD. As such, it does not, by definition at least, require close medical supervision. Slimfast is really no different from any of the other LCDs we have discussed, except it uses a liquid meal substitute (a shake) to control caloric intake.

The Slimfast diet plan involves consuming two of their shakes as a substitute for two meals each day. Often, another shake is taken as a snack. The other meal (usually supper) is a low-fat meal that you prepare. There are also low-calorie solid food snacks between meals.

I often recommend liquid meal substitution diets to my patients who aren't sure what debulking plan they want to try. My reasons include their low cost, ease of use, and relative safety. I like the fact that these plans do not require any meetings or supervision from often dubiously trained counselors. The Fat Madness Recovery Program is self-directed and designed to rebuild a sense of personal effectiveness. You don't need yet another expert to confuse the picture.

IT DOESN'T MATTER HOW YOU DO IT—JUST DO IT!

Any debulking plan can work. You can use a diet product, you can drink a shake, you can cut your portions, or eat food prepared for you by a genius chef who doesn't ever touch heavy cream or red meat. You can do anything healthy that involves lower caloric and fat intake and you will shed pounds.

However, none of these programs offers The Answer. It is up to you to use your decision-making power. Choose a plan that can help you, rather than be used by one that encourages you to become a member of their particular revolving door club. You now have the opportunity to feel a sense of coming recovery. You don't have to respond to every ad on television for that magic weight-loss-chocolate-bar program, or the diet pills, or the clever exercise machine that promises to relieve you of all your cellulite overnight.

None of the programs out there will truly help you maintain your weight loss, and none will teach you to recover from Fat Madness. This is your biggest job and the one that you must tackle after the pounds come off.

Don't buy into any promises that the moment you become a lifetime member of some plan, you will automatically be thin for the rest of your life. Use a diet program *only* for what it gives you in terms of weight loss goals and help coping with deprivation during debulking; don't be used by it in hopes of getting rewards in return for great expenditures of time and money.

What you want to do here is empower yourself to lose the weight. Don't go to a group like a sheep in a herd and listen to the same old pat concepts you've heard as long as you've been losing weight. Group support is fine in its place, and it's good to know there are others out there with your problem who share your concerns and can encourage you to achieve greater success.

But none of these offer any panacea, and even the die-hard converts to the programs keep coming back because they're hooked on their Fat Madness. They have to come back. They've gained back the weight they lost on this very plan.

Take the meetings and counseling for what they're worth, but don't rely on them. Rely only on yourself. You are the one who's been on and off the diet wagon all your life, and you're the one who's going to finally lick it.

These programs all offer different ways to cope with deprivation and give you help in denying yourself the foods you want. They give you tools to craft your own debulking process. They are not magic potions or powders, nor do they supply an end to your problem with weight control. The program coordinators will try to sell you motivational tapes, T-shirts, and coffee mugs. Remember, these programs can be expensive, and you don't want to add to your stress by giving yourself a financial as well as a dieting headache.

What are the alternatives to having your hand held in a program? You can save yourself a lot of bucks by buying a food-exchange cookbook recommended by your doctor or by going to your supermarket and using a combination of liquid shakes like Slimfast with good old homemade meals. There are excellent frozen dietary dinners and low-calorie meals you can select. Be sure to check the labels on the boxes to see that they're not too high in fat or sodium. You can also consult a registered dietician, who will customize meal plans for you and really teach you how to eat.

Then there's the ever-controversial issue of diet pills. The newest batch include fenfluramine (Pondimin) and phentermine (Fastin), two products that have many obesity researchers dancing jigs of excitement. Should you try them? This is a matter you must discuss with a reliable physician you know and trust. Diet pills have been around forever, and although they may assist in weight loss, they cannot keep the weight off.

Debulking is an artificial experience, so it's okay to use artificial means to achieve your goal. It's a temporary state of affairs and you can get the whole thing behind you within a six-month to one-year period, depending on the number of unhealthy pounds you're still carrying around. Please keep in mind, however, that when it's over, if you're still measuring, weighing, and evaluating food because you're scared you'll gain your weight back if you don't, you are obsessing and eventually will gain it all back.

How Strict Should You Be
with Your Debulking Program?

Can't you ever cheat? Just a little? Certainly you can, and it's crazy to think that you won't. However, I counsel you to be as religiously on target as you can be with whatever plan you choose, because you'll get it done faster. The sooner you get rid of the bulk, the sooner you can move on to a more liberal, natural, and normal eating style, which we'll discuss in Step 6.

If you decide, after reading through this step, that you simply cannot tolerate any more deprivation, if you're sick and tired of the rules and regulations about what you put in your mouth, then don't do it. Skip to Step 6 and start up your sane eating and exercise program today. Progress forward in your life instead of backward.

You can do it. You've gotten to this point in your recovery program, and you know that it's possible. Take a deep breath and turn the page, because it's time to start truly changing.

I Understand That Lasting Success Requires True Change

You are in a small boat in the ocean. You've been there for a long time. There is no horizon in sight.

Sometimes, it's terrifying. The idea of floating on and on, maybe forever, nearly paralyzes you. You feel so small and insignificant in this vast emptiness, totally impotent against wind and rain, against the staggering task of getting across all this water.

Other times, you feel resigned. It's okay, you'll make it. You've gotten this far, and with some good luck, you should make it through another night. If you don't waste your energies, if you just pray, it'll take care of itself.

But it seems to be completely in the hands of destiny. You feel powerless. The sea feels mammoth, much bigger than it really is.

Stop! This is madness, as you already know. Lasting success—the ability not only to survive but to reach your goal—requires true change. There is a motor on your boat; there is a bailing can. There's a lot of excess baggage you can dump overboard.

You make your fingers move and pull the starter rope, once, twice, and finally on the third try, it catches. You leave yourself just enough provisions and chuck everything else over the side. You take your can and start to bail.

You hit the horizon before nightfall. You made it.

Why Is Maintenance Like a Sea Voyage?

Life is like this. It's made of so many elements, and if you stop to look at them closely, you will be amazed at their similarities.

Being stuck in a boat is like dieting and losing weight and gaining it all over again because you think you can't change your behavior. How many times have you been able to maintain for weeks or months, but then fell off the wagon because your boss looked at you cross-eyed, or the tulips didn't come up, or you ended a passionate affair? For some reason—or no reason— you slumped back into the belief that nothing you could do would make a difference. You simply weren't able to incorporate those changes permanently into your behavior and thinking.

Probably you weren't ready then. Nobody really likes change; it's much more comfortable to do things the same old way. It takes guts and gumption to dare to be different. Maybe now, after all those dips and lulls, after watching the tides go in and out, you are ready for true change.

True change means you must look at your goals and see them, not as some vague point on the horizon or number on the scale or clothes rack, but as a lasting desire for more physical exercise and a better adaptation toward eating. The biggest change must be your acceptance of your own body, but we'll get to that in the final steps of the program.

Eating Is Not an Addiction

I want to stop and point out how the dieter is substantially different from the addict. The addict has a constant desire to please himself. He'll do anything for a high so he can feel great. In recovery, he must learn to turn around and give up something he wants to become more outward-oriented, more in touch with the world. The dieter, on the other hand, is always ready to please people. You know how many times you've claimed that you have to lose the weight for your husband or kids, that you have to look good so you can get that new job or go to your best friend's wedding.

For a dieter, true and lasting change in relation to food comes only when you begin to please yourself. It's not about looking good, but *feeling good*. This is not to say that you should abandon the concept of being attractive; only that you should start to recognize that attractiveness is relative to whomever is looking at you. And you, in your mirror, are the first viewer.

All right, you've debulked. That ought to tell you something about your opinion of yourself. You had the guts to do it one last time (or you were able to tell yourself you didn't need to do it, so you skipped that step and are already onto maintaining). Before, you had to have the outside world tell you that you were attractive. Now, you can rely on your inner resources.

As we've said, debulking is an unnatural, artificial experience that you can endure only for a limited amount of time without screaming, running away from home, or inhaling the entire gourmet section of your supermarket. The regimentation of eating that a debulking plan requires cannot be sustained over the long haul, nor should it be. It's time to liberalize your thinking about yourself, and your eating as well.

New Goals, New Horizons

Your new goal is to maximize your health and your inner feelings of well-being and to minimize your concerns about your external appearance. Okay, you aren't going to stop worrying about your thighs and butt overnight, but maybe now you're more awake and aware of their *relative* importance in your life. If you are gaining control over your Fat Madness, you are probably able to understand that you can't totally reshape your body (see Step 2 again if you have any doubts in that quarter).

But what you *can* do is reshape your health and feelings of worth. You can even do it at the expense of your scale. I have a patient named Harry who didn't lose a pound. As a matter of fact, he gained about five pounds during the time he was seeing me. And he never felt better. Why?

Because on his thirty-fifth birthday, sagging and out of breath, and terrified of having a massive coronary, he got up off his butt and started jogging. Every day, painful as it was at first, he made himself set the alarm for 6:30 and pop out of bed. (Well, maybe he didn't pop, but he made sure he threw off the covers.) He started walking four-tenths of a mile and worked his way up, over a four-year period, to complete a twenty-six-mile marathon. He dropped two inches on his waistline, got his blood pressure way down, and—since he also modified his diet—reduced his cholesterol level and triglycerides to the bottom of his normal range.

Harry is a happy man. He's fit and loves to exercise. He has changed the way he eats, the amount of time it takes him to consume his meals, and he eats a much wider variety of foods.

You can do this, too. Debulking, as we've said before, is really just a tool to help you think more about the enormous possibilities your body offers you. Only your mind will allow you to keep the weight off sanely, without depriving yourself, monitoring yourself, or driving yourself bananas.

The Road to Healthy Maintenance

You are the boss. Always remember this. Every diet program you've ever been on has made you slavishly obey some external authority. You have never before dealt with your internal management of food in relation to your world.

Real life demands that you learn to live with food. If you're going to stay at a healthy weight and be rid of your Fat Madness forever, you will have to do something about your old food preferences. No food plan in the world that involves measurement and deprivation can work for you long-term. That goes for any lack of plan that allows you to eat with mindless abandon.

Now you know enough about yourself to see that there are many facets involved here.

- You must learn to live with free-range food in a free-range world. You cannot continue to restrict your eating and deny yourself the bounty of what's out there. Restricted eating always sets you up for rebellion; you have to act out against restriction and eat your way through the supermarket, your house, and 7-Eleven.
- You have to use hunger and satiety as your guides. If you're in a healthy weight range, you will be eating everything and anything, but in appropriate amounts at appropriate times.
- You have to educate yourself on how to eat right. You can do this in any way you like. We offer the USDA Food Pyramid (see p. 138) as a useful tool.
- You have to explore other avenues of eating. There are plenty of grains, vegetables, fruits, and other low-fat delights you've probably never considered. Now's the time to taste, relish, and enjoy new foods.
- You have to move around. Daily exercise will be the real turning point in your maintenance program.

A New Consideration of Food

Let's forget what the media promises about delicious, mouth-watering, creamy, crunchy, delectable, betcha-can't-eat-just-one foods. The immediate taste in your mouth is over as soon as you swallow. One-dimensional. The quick fix. Nothing, in the great scheme of things.

We are now going to eat in three dimensions. The dimensions of your new food appreciation universe are:

Feelings.   You are going to choose foods that make you feel good not just as you taste them, but *after* you eat them. Hunger and satiety will tell you when to eat and when to stop.

Do the following experiment: Eat a fast-food cheeseburger with a bag of greasy chips and wash it down with a chocolate shake. Yes, it's okay, this is in the interests of science. Go back to your food diary and write down exactly how you felt after this meal. Stuffed, right? A meal filled with fat gives you a leaden, tired, uncomfortable feeling, makes you want to open your belt, lie down, and conk out.

Wait until you are hungry again. Then have a reasonable portion of pasta with red sauce, accompanied by a green salad and a roll, and wash them down with water or a sparkling fruit drink. Now, how do you feel? The complex carbohydrates, grains, and vegetables give you an up, energetic, alive feeling afterward. You are satiated rather than full.

Knowledge.   Let the USDA's food pyramid on page 138 guide you about how to balance the foods you should be considering on a daily maintenance program. This excellent chart will teach you most of what you have to know about nutrition by emphasizing the foods at the bottom (these you load up on) and glancing over the ones on top (these you eat minimally). The *American Heart Association Cookbook*, many low-fat ethnic cookbooks, and vegetarian cookbooks on the matter can be your guide to maximize health, increase your longevity, and prevent disease.

Behavior.   To alter the types and amounts of foods you select, you must first *expose* yourself to new foods, *substitute* healthy foods for those that aren't so good for you, and learn to control your *portions.*

Exposure only comes if you're willing to venture into unknown realms. You may not love Thai garlic parsley at first, but it could grow on you. You only know if you try it a few times with an open mind. You can reshape your food preferences by experimenting with new cuisines in new restaurants and venturing down aisles in the market that you previously ignored. So you never cooked kale. How hard could it be? Same for quinoa and amaranth. If you don't even know what these foods look like, ask at customer service. You may be astounded at some of the new taste sensations that are in store for you.

Substitution will happen over time. As you grow to love pasta, rice, vegetables, legumes, and whole-grain breads and cereals, they will become the staples of your diet. Fish, chicken, and lean beef will provide flavorings, something like condiments. You'll save money and learn to cook differently. And you will learn to automatically substitute low-fat alternatives (their number and quality is always growing) for all of the fat-filled foods you used to think you just had to have. The family will get used to it. Honest. If they don't, tough. This is *your* life.

Portion control is a necessary part of a good maintenance program, but now that you're eating from hunger and stopping because you're satiated, you may not have the problem with this that you anticipate.

Reality says that you're going to be eating better, but you'll also want to incorporate some of your old favorites into your diet as well. Old favorites are probably calorically dense, fat-filled foods. You can still eat them, as long as you eat them in reasonable amounts. By allowing yourself access to all foods and by following your new guidelines about eating only until you feel comfortable, you'll begin to limit your intake of sweets, fried foods, and other questionable items out of choice, not because you're supposed to.

It's Not All in the Food You Eat

When you make changes in your eating, you take a quantum leap toward recovery. Now that you're less obsessive about your caloric intake, you have the time to do something concrete and useful to improve your maintenance.

As a matter of fact, whether you've done anything radical about your eating or not, this extraordinary secret ingredient is going to do the job almost on its own.

The secret ingredient is called exercise. It is not called *exhaustion, overdoing*, or *fitness frenzy*, just plain old moving in space, allowing your body to explore the wonderful world of activity.

We haven't recommended an exercise program until this point because recovery is a one-step-at-a-time affair. If you tackle too much all at once, you risk disappointment. If you can't handle

The Food Guide Pyramid
A Guide to Daily Food Choices

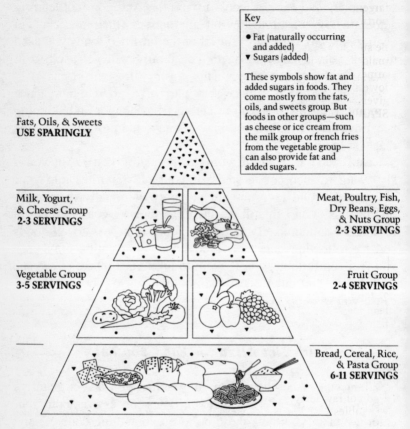

Key

- Fat (naturally occurring and added)
- ▼ Sugars (added)

These symbols show fat and added sugars in foods. They come mostly from the fats, oils, and sweets group. But foods in other groups—such as cheese or ice cream from the milk group or french fries from the vegetable group—can also provide fat and added sugars.

Fats, Oils, & Sweets
USE SPARINGLY

Milk, Yogurt, & Cheese Group
2-3 SERVINGS

Meat, Poultry, Fish, Dry Beans, Eggs, & Nuts Group
2-3 SERVINGS

Vegetable Group
3-5 SERVINGS

Fruit Group
2-4 SERVINGS

Bread, Cereal, Rice, & Pasta Group
6-11 SERVINGS

Looking at the Pieces of the Pyramid

The Food Guide Pyramid emphasizes foods from the five major food groups shown in the three lower sections of the Pyramid. Each of these food groups provides some, but not all, of the nutrients you need. Foods in one group can't replace those in another. No one of these major food groups is more important than another—for good health, you need them all.

Source: The United States Department of Agriculture

What Counts as 1 Serving?

The amount of food that counts as 1 serving is listed below. If you eat a larger portion, count it as more than 1 serving. For example, a dinner portion of spaghetti would count as 2 or 3 servings of pasta.

Be sure to eat at least the lowest number of servings from the five major food groups listed below. You need them for the vitamins, minerals, carbohydrates, and protein they provide. Just try to pick the lowest fat choices from the food groups. No specific serving size is given for the fats, oils, and sweets group because the message is USE SPARINGLY.

Food Groups

Milk, Yogurt, and Cheese		
1 cup of milk or yogurt	1½ ounces of natural cheese	2 ounces of process cheese

Meat, Poultry, Fish, Dry Beans, Eggs, and Nuts	
2–3 ounces of cooked lean meat, poultry, or fish	1/2 cup of cooked dry beans, 1 egg, or 2 tablespoons of peanut butter count as 1 ounce of lean meat

Vegetable		
1 cup of raw leafy vegetables	1/2 cup of other vegetables, cooked or chopped raw	3/4 cup of vegetable juice

Fruit		
1 medium apple, banana, orange	1/2 cup of chopped, cooked, or canned fruit	3/4 cup of fruit juice

Bread, Cereal, Rice, and Pasta		
1 slice of bread	1 ounce of ready-to-eat cereal	1/2 cup of cooked cereal, rice, or pasta

deprivation as you debulk along with having to get up twenty
minutes earlier for your walking program, you will end up feeling even more frustrated and upset with yourself. There's plenty
of time—your whole life, in fact—to work on your maintenance.
Why rush things?

This is the time to launch your exercise plan. Launch it and
let the wind take its sails and lift you from the lethargy of heavy
couch-potatodom to the buoyancy of feeling fit. This is not just
a poetic turn of phrase, it's the hard, cold truth: Exercise matters!
Of the few people who do successfully maintain a weight loss,
90 percent exercise regularly. They can liberalize their eating
because of the calories they burn moving around.

Why Exercise Is Good for You

You are the expert—you know that exercise is healthy from
your countless other weight-loss programs. But the elements are
worth repeating now, when they can really mean something new
to you. The benefits of regular exercise are surely more valuable
when you use them for true change. Exercise burns calories,
lowers your risk of heart disease and certain cancers, lowers your
stress level, improves your lung capacity, increases cardiovascular function, increases muscle strength, lowers LDL (bad) cholesterol and raises HDL (good) cholesterol, lowers serum
triglycerides, lowers blood sugar levels, keeps your bones strong
and joints flexible and helps to protect against arthritis and osteoporosis, improves your balance so it lowers your risk of ac-
cidental falls and injuries, regulates bowel function, lets you
sleep well at night, lowers depression and fatigue levels, and
enhances your appearance. And if all these reasons aren't
enough, it also improves your self-esteem and gives you an out-
let for social contact with other exercisers.

How Exercise and Good Nutrition Dovetail

Success breeds success. The more you exercise, the better you
feel, and the better you feel, the more you want to stick to your

excellent nutrition plan and get some more exercise. Conscious good health habits—not obsessive ones—become part of an inevitable cycle, like the waxing and waning of the tides and moon.

No, it does *not* make you hungrier if you move around. In fact, you feel less hungry because your body is using its fuel properly when it feeds its calories directly into energy consumption. It makes you feel particularly good if your diet is heavy on the complex carbohydrates, the macronutrient the body uses first for fuel (see Step 2 if you're fuzzy on this point).

Exercise helps you control your weight by reducing your appetite and burning off calories as you move, but it does more than that. It also indirectly influences the way your body processes foods and uses them for energy. This is done by increasing your basal metabolic rate so that you actually continue to burn calories after exercise, *when your body is at rest*. Yes, it's true. You'd not only burn 300 calories on a brisk two-mile walk, you'd also keep burning calories faster afterward, as you sat at your computer or sorted the laundry.

See how this can affect what you eat? After you've gotten to your goal weight, if you're exercising daily, you can begin to increase the amounts of healthy food in your diet and not gain a pound.

Remember, too, that exercise builds muscle, and muscle tissue burns more calories than fat tissue, even when those muscles are at rest. So as you build muscle mass through your workouts, you increase your body's energy expenditure, and can therefore afford to consume a bag of chips or a slice of cake every once in a while.

How to Do This Wonderful Thing Called Exercise

Let's break it down and make it really simple. Just remember that before beginning *any* of these plans, you need your physician's okay and you should own a good pair of exercise shoes.

The Three-Option Exercise Plan

OPTION 1. Increase physical activity in your daily life.
OPTION 2. Start a walking program.
OPTION 3. Practice the Exercise Exchange.

Everyone has his or her excuses about not exercising. But it isn't true that everyone's too busy, bored, or injured to keep on track with a calm and comfortable daily exercise regimen. Nor should you stoop to the excuse that if your family and friends don't support you in this endeavor, it's just impossible. After all, you debulked on your own, so you can exercise on your own.

The best way to stick with an activity program is to find something you really like to do. If you've tried and failed before, you ought to start with the most basic of the three exercise options.

Option 1: Increase Physical Activity in Your Daily Life

Right now, you say you can't get up earlier, you can't go to bed later, you can't afford a gym, and you aren't near a pool. Let us assume that at the moment that this is true. You can't begin a formal program. You can, however, take all the things that you ordinarily do and add a calorie-burning component to them.

Option 1 enables you to increase your level of daily activity in an informal, unstructured way. It will contribute to weight control and should add a different dimension to your days. If you wish to lose more weight than you have on your debulking plan thus far, you'll have to move onto Option 2 or 3 so that you are actually burning 1,500 to 3,000 calories a week. However, stick with this option until you feel you've mastered it and are ready for a bigger challenge.

Let's look at the subtle but significant ways you can change the way you do the things you do.

Transportation. Change the way you get around. This will take a little brain work, but here are some suggestions.

- Walk or ride a bike instead of driving to work or school.
- Park farther from your destination and walk more.
- Walk, don't drive, to the mailbox, and, if your location permits, to the newsstand and the convenience store.
- In the mall, walk up and down the escalators.
- In an elevator building, take the stairs whenever fire laws permit.

At home. Remember, every calorie burned is another step in your maintenance plan. Here are a few suggestions.

- Put away your television remote control. Get up to change channels.
- Don't ever sit passively in front of the television. Even if it's just for a few minutes, jog in place, do some slow stretches, or keep a piece of exercise equipment, like a stationary bike, a treadmill, or a rowing machine in the room to use as you watch.
- Wash the car (and the dog) yourself.
- If you are bored, get up and walk around the block.
- When you clean the house, do one room on the first floor, then one on the second, then one on the first, etc.
- Walk the dog at a nice, brisk pace (good for the dog, too!).
- Do a big cleaning or home maintenance job every few weeks: wash the windows; clean the attic, basement, garage, or closets. Work to music with a lively beat so you'll move faster.
- Do some yard work every week: pull weeds, sweep the walk, rake leaves, etc. Again, work to music.

Leisure activities. Instead of sitting around the house reading or watching television, you could be out doing things that burn calories. For example:

- Hit a tennis ball against the wall.
- Shoot baskets.
- Go out dancing with your spouse or partner.
- Go bowling.
- Ride a bike.
- Go ice skating with your kids.

How many calories is this really going to burn? It doesn't matter. Don't even count them. It is not the numbers we're thinking of here, but changing your routine. Just add some physical activity to your daily life. There's a real good chance that you'll want to move onto a more formal exercise plan once you get used to doing more with your body. It can only do you good.

A study at Stanford University on 17,000 Harvard graduates showed that those who burned in excess of 2,000 calories a week (for an individual who weighs 140, that's about the equivalent of walking an hour each day) had a 28 percent lower all-cause death rate than those who were less active. And these people didn't just live longer because they were fit. They also liked themselves and were psychologically in better shape than those who just sat around doing nothing but worrying about their weight. It has been clearly documented that any form of exercise raises the level of beta endorphins in your brain, those polypeptides that act as natural opiates, making you feel great.

Option 2: The Walking Program

Our evolution into human beings occurred when our ancestors made the decision to stand up on their hind legs. This upright position allows us, as it did those who came before us, the unique privilege of seeing the whole world as we move in it. How lucky we are to be able to walk!

You don't have to learn anything new. You've been walking since you were knee-high to the television set, so you're pretty much an expert at it. You need no special equipment other than a comfortable pair of shoes. These don't have to be dedicated walking shoes, all they must do is fit well and have thick, flexible soles that can cushion the impact of your feet hitting the ground.

You can walk alone, with a spouse or friend, or in a pack. You can walk slowly or fast or (even better) alternate your rhythms. You can wear a headset and walk to the news or music or a tape of the latest best-selling novel. Just make sure the volume isn't so loud that you can't hear car horns.

You can walk inside at a track in a health club or gym, or in a mall. (There are often groups that mall-walk in the early morning so you can window-shop at the same time.) You can walk everywhere and anywhere outside. You can go down the block, out into the country, or around a track at the local high school. Wear light, loose-fitting clothes, and dress in layers so that you can start to peel clothes off when you get warmed up. If you have started with Option 1, you may have purchased a treadmill for your television room, in which case you can walk all by yourself at home.

Start slowly and build up your pace gradually. Don't worry about burning calories—there will be time for that later. The important thing is to build your stamina and endurance in a progressive, healthful manner. This way you won't suffer from shin splints, blisters, or other injuries.

Plan to walk at least three days a week to start, then build up gradually to six or seven days over a period of four weeks. Set a pace that would allow you to talk to a friend without gasping for breath. If you miss a planned walk, that's okay. Just reschedule your walk for later that day or the next day. Cut back to a slower pace if you're tired or sore.

As soon as you're comfortable at a slow pace, increase your speed a little. Here are some tips on the advanced walking program, which you should be able to achieve over a period of about eight weeks:

· Walk at a brisk pace of about four miles an hour.
· Carry light (one- to three-pound) weights in each hand and swing them rhythmically as you walk. Don't use the weights

that strap onto your wrists, as they can injure tendons and interfere with circulation.
- Choose a route that includes going up and down hills.
- Eventually, move your pace up to four and a half miles an hour.

Warning Signs That You Are Exercising Incorrectly

Some mild aches and pains are to be expected, particularly if you've been sitting on your duff for years, but if you hurt all the time, something's wrong. Persistent pain and soreness means that you are pushing yourself too hard, forgetting to breathe properly as you move (more common than you might imagine), or that you have some chronic ailment that's being exacerbated by the new energy put forth by your body.

You may wish to consult your physician or a trainer at your local Y or health club if you are in doubt about how serious an injury might be.

Stop exercising and see a doctor immediately if you have squeezing or crushing chest pain, whether you are a man or a woman. The same advice applies if you become dizzy or light-headed or have trouble catching your breath.

Option 3: The Exercise Exchange Program

If you are really ready for the pleasures of exercise, you will want to move on from walking (not abandoning this activity, just adding to it). An aerobic program that gets you to reach a training level suitable to your age will make your heart beat faster, your lungs work harder, your muscles expand and improve, and will get you to sweat. (Sweat is nice. It is your body's way of releasing the new energy you're expending.)

The Exercise Exchange Program will allow you to burn 1,500 to 3,000 calories a week. It's called an exchange, just like that kind of diet, because you can substitute energy-equivalent activities for greater variety. Certain of these exchanges burn lots of calories, others significantly less. Again, don't bother counting. It's the doing that's important.

Activity	Calorie Burning Level
Slow jogging	Medium
Running	High
Swimming	Medium
Cycling	Medium
Racquet sports (tennis, squash, racquetball)	High
Team sports (basketball, hockey, soccer)	Medium
Aerobic dancing	High
Step-training	High
Ice-skating and roller-blading	Medium
Cross-country skiing	High
Downhill skiing	Medium
Martial arts	Medium
Exercise machines	High

When you mix and match your exercise programs, you are *cross-training*. This means you are using different muscle groups, and the end result is that all of you gets trained at some time during the week. Your entire body becomes stronger and better conditioned when you complement one type of activity with another. An aerobic activity like running will give you stamina and endurance as well as lower-body strength. Swimming is aerobic, though not weight bearing, so although it won't do much for the strength of your bones, it will work wonders on your lung capacity and upper-body strength. Martial arts will work on your balance and flexibility as well as develop quick reflexes and inner energy.

When you look down the list of activities above, you'll see some items you already enjoy and others that you may have always had a yen to try. Go ahead! Be daring! The following suggestions will help you get started:

- Sign up for a ten-week course in a Y or community education program. This doesn't represent an enormous commitment of time or money and will allow you to sample a few choices.
- Beware of health-club lifetime memberships, which can be a waste of big bucks if you drop out.
- If you like competitive sports, set up a weekly game with a partner who's at your level or a little more skillful than you. You'll be less likely to skip your exercise session if you know that someone else is depending on you to be there.
- Set aside at least sixty minutes (including warm-up and cool-down) for one session of whatever sport you participate in.
- Aim for a minimum of four workouts per week.

Aerobic Conditioning

The kind of exercise that gets your heart pounding, your lungs expanding, and your body sweating buckets is *aerobic,* because it uses all your inspiration (the air you take in) to perform it. As you get better at aerobic exercise, it increases the efficiency of oxygen intake to your body, gives you endurance for more exercise and incidentally, as it strengthens and improves the muscle that is your heart, protects you against coronary artery disease.

To get good at this stuff, you need at least four thirty-minute aerobic workouts a week at a level that's intense enough to raise your heart rate to your appropriate *training rate,* or the rate at which your heart should be beating during strenuous exercise.

You can learn how hard your heart should be working by figuring out the difference between your *resting heart rate* (when you're sitting quietly in a chair) and your *maximum heart rate* (the very fastest your heart could pump, given your age). You never actually want to get your heart rate up to the maximum; it would be very dangerous.

The way you compute your training heart rate is by subtracting your age from 220, then multiplying by 60 percent of your maximum rate (you may go up to 70 percent if you're in training for an athletic competition). You can wear a fancy gizmo from a sporting goods store, which will beep when you hit your training heart rate, but it's easier to keep your fingers on your pulse at the carotid artery on the side of your neck while you're jogging or pedaling your bike uphill. Count the beats for ten seconds and multiply the results by six.

Don't expect to hit your rate your first time out. Remember, your body must get used to the new demands you're putting on it. As you get better, you'll find that you achieve your training rate more quickly and efficiently.

If you don't want to take your hand off the handlebars to take your pulse, you can also find out how you're doing by using another method, called the *rating of perceived exertion*. In this system, you rate yourself as exercising at a pace that's very easy, very difficult, or somewhere in between. You should get that correct in-between feeling if you are barely able to carry on a conversation with someone while exercising. If you've got plenty of air to talk, you're not working hard enough. If you're huffing and puffing and can scarcely choke out a word, you're working too hard.

Warming Up and Cooling Down

After our teen years, regardless of age or fitness level, we are all creaky when we wake up in the morning or after having been sedentary all day, so we all need some preparation for exercise. Without some basic warm-ups, we can't really commit our bodies to the exercise we want to do. More important, we want to avoid injuries and prevent strain on the cardiovascular system. Warming up comes in two parts:

Warm-up I—Stretching

When you make physical demands on your muscles, they have to contract and elongate more quickly. If they aren't warm, their fibers aren't properly loosened so that they can really move.

Spend between five and ten minutes doing the following stretching exercises.

Neck rolls. Drop your chin onto your chest and slowly roll your head to the right, then back to center, then left. Proceed to rolling in a complete circle, trying to get your ear to your shoulder as you come around. Reverse the circle.

Shoulder rolls. Relax your arms and drop your shoulders. Then rotate your right shoulder in a full circle three times, trying to touch your ear with your shoulder. Repeat on the left side. Then rotate both shoulders together in the same direction three times, then with one shoulder going forward and the other backward three times. Reverse.

Side stretch. Stand with your feet apart, knees slightly bent. Extend your right arm over your head while leaning your trunk as far as you can to the left; then do the same with your left arm as you lean to the right. Be sure to keep your body facing straight ahead as you bend to the sides. Repeat three times on each side.

Lower body stretch. Lie on your back on the floor and pull one knee up to your chest, then the other. After three repetitions on each side, pull both knees to your chest, wrap your arms around them, and rock back and forth. Think about sinking your waist into the floor.

Back and leg stretches. Sit on the floor and spread your legs in a V. Straighten your knees if you can, but it's more important to stay upright. Reach for the toes of the right foot with both hands and pull yourself to the right, trying to put your nose on your knee; do the same to the left. Come up slowly. Repeat three times on each side.

Calf stretch. Stand up and place your right foot flat on the floor in front of your body, putting the weight on it as you bend your right knee. Straighten the back leg, keeping your back straight, as you lean into your right quadricep (the big muscle on top of your thigh). Hold it for a count of ten. Repeat three times on each side.

Warm-up II—Build Up Pace to Training Rate

Spend five to ten minutes at this warm-up. If you're going to jog, start out at a walk and gradually increase your pace over a five-minute interval. You may alternately walk and jog at an easy rate after that until you are finally just jogging. If you are biking, start on the flats and pedal on the lowest gear for five minutes; gradually increase the tension as you work your way up to your training rate.

If you exercise at a Y or a gym on machines, ask your instructor to lead you through a warm-up. (Any reputable step-training and low-impact aerobic class will have this built into their routines.) If you're working on machines, they usually have a warm-up built into their programs, too.

The *cool-down* phase, after your exercise workout, is just as important as the warm-up. You want to get your body back to its regular slow pace gradually and lower your heart rate. If you don't, painful cramps may result. A good cool-down may prevent next-day soreness after a particularly strenuous workout.

If you're jogging, gradually start to slow your pace until you reach a walk. If you're biking, get back down to a low gear. In a class of any sort, work more slowly and do exercises that require less effort.

You're cooling down properly when your pulse is back at its resting rate within five minutes of reducing the intensity of your workout.

Ideally, for a complete cycle, you should once again perform your warm-up exercises.

Anaerobic Conditioning Helps You Maintain True Change

Your exercise menu wouldn't be complete without one other element: *anaerobic conditioning*. This type of activity raises your pulse rate but is not intended for sustained periods of cardiovascular work, as aerobic exercise is. Instead, it's intended to increase the mass and/or strength of certain muscle groups.

Weight-lifting is a good example of this type of activity. You probably won't shed pounds lifting, but you will tone and condition your body. Weight-lifting builds metabolically active tissue (muscle tissue) and allows you to eat more and still not gain weight.

Running and cycling are great, but they won't do much for your upper body. In order to have a good balance of fitness, you also need to strengthen your arm and chest muscles.

You must have instruction if you're going to do weight training, which will mean joining a Y or a health club. Your trainer will show you how to work up to a certain number of reps (repetitions) on each piece of equipment.

Circuit training. In this type of resistance training, you push or pull against the resistance offered by certain machines. You work out on one machine, usually part of a Nautilus or Lifecircuit system, then move to the next. Trainers customize particular programs for their clients, depending on their needs.

Free weights. You work out by lifting weights you can hold in your hand. Many repetitions with lighter weights build strength. Fewer repetitions with heavier weights build muscle mass.

When to Exercise

The argument rages over whether it's better to exercise in the morning, night, or at midday. Actually, *it's best to exercise whenever you're willing to do it.* If you have no particular preferences, here are some thoughts that might make you adjust your exercise clock.

Morning. All you have to do is get up half an hour earlier. Many people find that it's easier to concentrate and breathe before the hassles and upsets of a normal day have begun. Some people also find the morning to be a special personal time, when the kids and spouse are still asleep, the streets belong to you instead of the cars, and the sun is rising in all its glory.

Afternoon. If you devote your lunch hour to exercise, you don't have time to eat much. Exercise can also give you a head start on the typical 3:00 P.M. exhaustion syndrome, when most people experience a decrease in energy. If you work for a corporation with a gym and locker room or if you work at home, you don't have the concern of smelling like a goat for the rest of the day, either. If you're a homemaker and your kids are in school, this is a great time to give yourself a break when they're not around.

Evening. Evening exercise helps you to wind down after a long day. If you like to work out with others, this is probably the best time of day to find a partner. It can also keep you away from the temptation of midnight (or 9:00 P.M.) snacking. If you find that evening exercise gives you too much energy and you have trouble falling asleep, move the time up a little and exercise right after work, before dinner.

Make it a habit. At the beginning, use a calendar to make dates with yourself for exercise. If you miss a scheduled period, reschedule it immediately. You don't necessarily have to book yourself for the same time of day every day, but a similar weekly plan is a good idea so that you can begin to make exercise a habit. You know how hard it is to break a habit. so you might as well make positive ones as negative ones. The habit of exercise will become a fixture in your life in a couple of months, as impossible to get rid of as your Beatles record collection.

Feeling Good As a Component in Recovery

You really can achieve inner peace through exercise. This is not a lot of nonsense. Surely you have read accounts of great professional athletes who talk about The Flow. The basketball player who sees the hoop as a huge hammock and all the defensive guards as little ants; the tennis player who imagines her tennis ball growing to the size of beach ball so that she can't miss it when she swings. The sense of skillful accomplishment and the ability and ease of motion comprise the basics of The Flow. It's an experience we can all feel when we are in training. This can happen when our mind is totally in sync with our body and we harmonize with the space we inhabit.

It is vitally important to develop a *love* for the way exercise makes your body feel before, during, and after it; for the extra oomph it gives you during the day and at night; for the way it changes your body; for reminding you that we are all human and possess this amazing, facile, talented machine that functions well or badly, depending on the circumstances.

If you think exercise is boring, smelly, irritating, unpleasant, or just plain no fun, you need to change your attitude. The reason is that, no matter how radically you alter your food preferences and control your portions, your chances of maintaining your weight loss will be *drastically reduced* without the benefits of exercise, and your health just won't be as good. You'll still feel tired a lot of the time. You'll still be concentrating more on the food parts of this program than the overall approach to better living. So do it today. Fall in love. It may take a fancy new exercise outfit or a purple bike or a great tai chi teacher, but find a way to do it.

When you start an exercise regimen, you will begin to discover all sorts of innovative ways to change your behavior through your new achievements and habits. You won't have to worry about rules and regulations about eating or about missing one day in your walking program. The elements will miraculously come together on their own, in their own time.

Be Selfish About Your Goals

I'm going to ask something really radical. I am requesting that you be selfish when it comes to effecting your true change. Remember what I said before about the addict having problems giving up anything for others? The dieter is the flip side of this and usually does everything for other people. But it takes healthy selfishness to tell your family you can't make dinner right away because you're going for your evening bike ride. It takes self-ishness to insist that you want a vegetarian meal at least once a week, and if they choose not to partake, they must make their own food. It's certainly selfish to ask your friends to try out a low-cal Thai restaurant instead of the heavy-cream French one they always want to go to.

This is okay. You owe it to yourself to get rid of those pressures that have caused you to succumb to Fat Madness in the past. So what if society is all hung up on how you should party or what you should look like? You must realize that being selfish means your task of true change is so important that you can't deviate from it, nor can anyone else make you.

You are now really ensconced in your recovery, so I can tell you that you will never actually reach the goal you think you want to reach. You will always be moving toward it, but you'll never just wake up one day and say, "Well, I used to have a problem with food and my body, but it's gone now." It's always there to be worked on, but now your work will be enjoyable instead of arduous. You're never a recovered addict, after all, but always engaged in the process of recovering.

You have taken a giant step. Five steps ago, you didn't even know the questions that had to be asked about yourself and your worth and whether it was more important to make yourself miserable or fit into a size 6. You have to have progressed to this point in order to see even the possibilities of all those questions out there you still don't know how to ask. Don't look for answers yet. They'll come in time.

True change and recovery comes *after* the time when you think the work is done. Just a little while ago, you wouldn't have been ready to hear that. Now you are ready to alter your goals and ideals. You know you'll keep changing them all along the way as they fit better in your healthier approach to life.

Try New Things

You now have the power to shake yourself up, to get out of old habits and create new ones. You will start to think differently about eating and exercising once the gradual switch-over from old, familiar behaviors becomes more consistent with the way you feel—inside as well as out-side—about your body. When the new becomes common-place, it will be time to shake yourself up again. Change means progression; stagnation can be death.

Give these suggestions a try, and don't judge them until you've tried them *all*.

> Eat six small meals a day instead of three large ones.
> Don't eat at traditional meal hours, but only when you actually feel hungry.
> Keep some carrots, papaya, or a cantaloupe at the of-fice for an emergency food fix. These foods are filled with beta-carotene, which happens to be an antioxidant that may prevent you from getting heart disease or cancer.
> Move all the furniture out of one room or part of a room in your house or apartment and make it your exercise nook. When you're in that space, you *must* stretch, jog in place, meditate, or do some breathing.

Get friendly with your local health-food store owner and ask if he or she might consider giving you a discount in exchange for bringing in other customers or purchasing some bulk orders of foods such as rice, pasta, and grains.

Buy a wok and experiment with Eastern cooking. You can cook anything in a wok. Just stir-fry some vegetables and tofu and serve them over rice. Use a little beef or chicken for flavoring.

Try at least one new recipe per week. Keep notes as to how you liked it and why you would or wouldn't try it again. What is interesting about kidney beans? What is unusual about Japanese nori?

Pay attention to the diets your friends are on. When they talk about their obsessions with food or body image, think about how you used to express yourself on these issues. See how differently you feel now than you used to.

Find a friend or acquaintance who has run a marathon, participated in an athletic competition, or performed in a dance contest and find out how they got to the physical and mental state they're now in.

I Will No Longer Be a Victim

You're probably feeling pretty good about yourself right now, and if you've made it through the first six steps of your Fat Madness Recovery Program, you have every right to be pleased. You are probably either still debulking and looking forward to following your new maintenance plan, or you are working hard to incorporate the habits and behavior changes suggested in Step 6 into your life.

I bet you feel like you've finally found the answer to your lifelong battle with Fat Madness. You're filled with hope that, this time, it's going to work. This time, the old fears and panic about food and your body will never come creeping back out of the closet to get you, and you'll continue merrily on your maintenance program without a care in the world. Things will be bright and cheery. The end.

But wait. Remember what I said before? Life is not a finished product. Neither is a preoccupation with the way you look or the way you think others see you. Change is never all there or all *not* there because, of course, it's still changing.

You have been on many other diets, many other exercise programs, so you know that this is precisely the time when you start congratulating yourself and forget how you got where you are. You already know without having to be told that this is not the time to sit back and relax. In fact, this is the time to be even more vigilant. You have tasted success. You've proven to yourself that you do, in fact, have control over your eating and your exercising. You should relish this success because it can set the stage for the larger challenges to come.

You have changed your behavior, and that is a mammoth accomplishment. Now, you must work on changing your attitude and emotions, which is a much harder job. You have to alter your mentality so that your first reaction to a difficult situation is no longer "I can't" but "I can." Remember that neat kid's book, *The Little Engine That Could*? There was no way such a tiny piece of machinery was going to make it over the mountain by itself. Yet by repeating over and over, "I think I can, I think I can," the little engine completed the journey and ended up saying, "I *knew* I could."

You are that little engine. And you really *can* do it if you tackle the much more illusive and complex but very rewarding part of your recovery work. Now you are going to take the final steps to make sure you really have discovered a permanent solution to getting on and off the weight wagon.

Why This Is a Breakpoint Time in Your Recovery

Addictive behaviors—and that includes the behavior of eating obsessively and dieting and worrying so much about your body that you start eating obsessively again—can start up again. They may stay dormant for days, weeks, months, or even years after recovery, and then, suddenly, seemingly for no reason, they reappear fully blown, as though they never left you.

There is a reason. Most people never finish the work they must do to make true change a part of their lives. They just don't believe, deep down, that they deserve to do well. People who suffer from Fat Madness often find it difficult to accept success. Their inner programming to fail is so deeply embedded that success seems strange and uncomfortable.

Why should it feel wrong to do right by yourself? You've been fed a load of baloney about how imperfect you are and why you *should* change. You've been told that if only you had two inches less on your thighs, you'd be in the running to earn a million dollars and also be included on next year's Best Dressed list. You've been handed a bundle of impossible expectations and negative messages about your self-image throughout your life. How could it ever feel right to enjoy what you've accomplished this far and to believe that you can continue it?

So please stick with me. The last three steps of the Fat Madness Recovery Program are essential to your complete and full change of direction from self-doubt and self-loathing to liking yourself for yourself. They really can help you overcome those barriers to lasting achievement and serenity.

I think this is a very good time for a case history, and Angela represents to me one of the classic examples of why you can't stop with Step 6. When Angela came to see me, she was fed up with her life of yo-yo dieting. She was sick and tired of being preoccupied with her body. Angela was diligent about the Fat Madness Recovery Program, doing all of her recommended exercises, practicing hunger and satiety cues until they were second nature, and developing a personalized exercise plan she really liked and could stick with. The only thing she didn't do was follow through on Steps 7 to 9. She didn't feel she needed them.

When she came back to me a year after abandoning the program, she was desperate once again. I think it's worthwhile to repeat our conversation verbatim.

ANGELA: I just don't get it. After all that work and feeling so good about myself, how could I be binging on garbage again? I learned to like and respect my body. Now I'm starting to pick myself apart, just like I used to.

DR. SINAIKIN: Well, what exactly is going on in your head while you are *undoing* your program?

ANGELA: *(She smiles ruefully at the word I've just thrown out.)* I don't really know. It's an uneasy feeling. I don't feel good about myself even though I'm doing good things for myself.

DR. SINAIKIN: Can you pick up on a thought or event that made you start to feel bad?

ANGELA: *(She gives it a little reflection.)* Yes. I think I know. I was at a family reunion and my Aunt Beatrice commented that I looked pretty good but could stand to lose some weight in my legs. I don't know why that bothered me. I don't even like my Aunt Beatrice and believe me, *she* could stand to lose some weight from her whole body! But I guess that one nasty remark set off something in me, because I started to eat junk again the next day. A couple of weeks later, I started sloughing off on my exercise, and then the old tapes started playing. You know, that I'm fat and a failure. That kind of stuff.

DR. SINAIKIN: So just that one comment set you back?

ANGELA: Yeah, amazing as that seems. After all the work I did, one negative remark from my idiot aunt and it was Fat Madness all over again.

DR. SINAIKIN: Actually, that's not amazing at all. That's usually how it happens. *(I paused before asking the next question.)* So, does it feel more normal to be struggling with your weight issue again, being good one day and bad the next? Or did it feel more normal when you were succeeding?

ANGELA: *(She looks upset as she begins to understand exactly what's going on inside herself.)* I think—oh, God, I think that's it. It definitely feels more normal to be struggling. It's like I missed my Fat Madness and, even though I hate it, now that I have it back, it feels like I'm myself again.

Negative Self-Image Is the Killer

So this is the real problem: The deeply ingrained negative self-image and low self-esteem that Angela has battled all her life *is the norm*. It has been part of her so long that she cannot bear to live without it, even though she knows it's bad for her and it causes her to lapse right back into old self-destructive habits.

Angela isn't the only one who falls into this trap. If you don't work your way through the finishing steps of the recovery program, it can threaten to come back to haunt you at any time.

Notice that I didn't say "until you *finish* your recovery program." It is never finished. Just as an alcoholic never recovers, but is always in recovery, so a person afflicted with Fat Madness must always be on the alert for attitudes that can spring up once again and start the vicious cycle.

The problem Angela and everyone else on the program experiences is the very same problem we've been dealing with throughout the book. Why come back to it now, after all of the behavior and attitude changes we've already worked on? It's because now, with new habits and behavior already in place, you are in a far stronger emotional position than ever before. You need to feel this confident about yourself in order to conquer your Fat Madness at last. You can only do this from a position of strength.

The first step in that process is to learn how to undo the damage that has already been done to you.

Muddying Up the Brainwashing

The reason you succumbed to Fat Madness in the first place was because you were brainwashed by your family, society, the culture, the media. What exactly is brainwashing and how does it cause you to sabotage efforts to change, even when you really want to?

Brainwashing occurs when an outside force or influence causes you to view the world in a certain way, to develop a certain perspective of reality that actually becomes your reality. It is a brilliant, systematic programming of the human mind to alter it without the subject even being aware that a radical change has taken place. We tend to view brainwashing in a negative light, of course, because we associate it with evil captors and prisoners of war, and Patty Hearst locked in a closet.

But taken from a broader perspective, brainwashing can be seen as a pervasive phenomenon by which each culture or society teaches its members what life and the world means. There are hundreds of good examples of how brainwashing works. In our society, men don't wear dresses (unless they're having some gender confusion), but if you go to Scotland, you see that people don't look twice at a man in a kilt. Consider ants. We don't eat ants, but lots of tribes in Africa consider them an excellent source of protein. Just think about the times you have tried to understand the perspective of someone from a different cultural background. No matter how right you feel, the other person feels equally right in his or her view. In fact, you are right and so are they. Everyone's entitled to an opinion.

Is your Fat Madness a result of brainwashing? Let me offer another case history so we can examine this better.

Marion was a patient of mine who had a lot of negative feelings about her body and suffered terribly from low self-esteem. We tried to get at the sources of these feelings together. I asked her to recall the first time she remembered feeling ashamed of her body, and she immediately brought up what she considered her very first memory from childhood. Marion distinctly recalled the hurtful things her brother and his friends would say to her when she was four—that she was so huge, she'd break the chair. That she couldn't even fit on the toilet seat, and in a year, they'd have to make her a special one in blimp size. She had to go ask her mother what blimp meant.

Her sympathetic mother offered to help her by putting her on a diet. This resulted in Marion's first failed attempt to get thin. It also resulted in her perception that it was right to be ashamed of her body. By the time she reached kindergarten, she felt different from everyone else.

Despite having a wonderful, caring kindergarten teacher, Marion's problem got worse. The teacher thought she was helping Marion by offering her an apple instead of the graham crackers and milk the rest of the class was having. What this did was to reinforce Marion's feeling that she was an alien. Although the teacher attempted to stop the other kids from teasing Marion, they heard another message that reinforced their cruelty. The message was, "Marion's too fat to eat cookies."

Marion's Fat Madness was confirmed by what she saw on television. Her reality jibed with that of many characters on many of the shows. Chubby kids on television were teased just like she was teased in school. And the beautiful people on television were thin, happy, and smart. She also observed that her mother was always trying to get thin, via some new diet. So even when her mom tried to help her deal with her negative feelings, even when her mom tried to comfort her and make her feel better about herself, she knew that her mom was lying. She could see clearly that the only solution to her problem was to get thin.

And she did it. By denying herself food, she slimmed down by the time she got to junior high school. This still didn't make her happy, because she was too busy worrying about getting fat again. Besides, she knew that her body was far from perfect. The really popular girls were incredibly pretty (incredibly thin). This helped her to formulate a reason why she wasn't popular, and this gave her yet another message about how the game of life was played.

Once again, her mother tried to help Marion. She was always praising her for things Marion didn't care about at all, like her brains and her personality. It was like that old joke about the guys standing around and trying to think of something nice to say about the fat girl. ''Well, she's got a really good personality,'' one ventures after everyone's been racking his brain. The guys all guffaw loudly. As if that mattered!

Marion could see that it didn't matter, just by looking at her mother. If brains and personality were so important, then why was her mom always on a diet? The constant struggle to be thin was like a bad smell hanging over their house.

One day, Marion read an article in a magazine that explained how body weight is genetically determined and how, for some people, it is next to impossible to get down to a really low weight and stay there. Instead of reassuring Marion that there were elements here that were really out of her hands and she should get busy accepting the body she had, the article scared the hell out of her.

That was the day that Marion became anorexic. She was convinced that not eating at all was the only solution for her. It worked. She managed to starve herself down to ninety-two pounds. Yet she still felt fat.

By the time Marion became my patient, she had already had some excellent care that allowed her to see her anorexia as a symptom of her greater illness. She was stopped in her quest for perfection before she went too far and killed herself, but she was still struggling with her weight and self-esteem.

Marion came to see me because she still believed she was supposed to be thin. She was on a crazy turntable of dieting, depriving herself on one plan for a few days, then falling off, then trying another plan. She had completely burnt out on dieting, but she was more preoccupied with her Fat Madness than ever. Now she had a few new theories: Maybe it was her thyroid, or maybe it was chronic depression.

After we got past the practical work in Steps 1 to 6, Marion arrived at the crossroads. It was time for her to make permanent changes in her behavior and attitudes. She looked at me one day and acknowledged that she wasn't depressed, she wasn't hypothyroid. The only thing wrong with her, she had discovered, was a lifetime of brainwashing by Fat Madness. We needed to undo the brainwashing.

Getting Rid of Your Distorted Attitudes

Twenty or thirty years of brainwashing can't be cleared up overnight. There's a great deal of hard work to do as you discover the attitudes, thoughts, and beliefs you live by today. It doesn't really matter where these came from since you can't go back and change the past. The present, however, is another matter. When you know how your brainwashing expresses itself in the here and now, you are one step closer to defeating it.

We can attack the bad attitudes, thoughts, and beliefs you carry with you each day by *identifying them* and then *substituting rational ideas* in their place. But first we need to set the stage for this important work.

Change Comes When You Are Emotionally Ready for It

You can't get anywhere when you're stuck. If you deny all the feelings that make you miserable, self-doubting, and helpless, you're stuck but good!

Positive changes in distorted attitudes, thoughts, and beliefs only happen when you're in a receptive emotional state. I'm not suggesting that you just smile and sit back and hope that good feelings will land in your heart. The pleasant feelings don't always teach us what we have to learn about ourselves. Some of the emotions we don't like to feel, *anger* being the primary one, will put us in touch with what's going on.

Appropriate anger is one particularly terrific emotion that lets us get rid of self-hating feelings, especially when it's expressed as righteous indignation. This feeling gives you the energy you will need to fuel the changes you're going to make. Anger is necessary to help you ward off new brainwashing forces that will be working to sabotage your efforts to change.

Anger Can Be Good for You

Anger is the appropriate emotional response if you're being victimized. If you're a kid on your way to school and some big bully takes your allowance money, *you have every right to be angry*. If you're an excellent worker, and someone else gets the promotion you wanted, *why shouldn't you feel like you've been abused?* You need to see that your Fat Madness brainwashing is abuse and victimization by an unfeeling and cruel culture.

You are very well aware from Step 2 that your body weight and especially your body shape are primarily genetically determined, yet for your whole life, you've been made to feel personally responsible for something that is basically out of your control. If you'd ever been attacked because of your height or skin color, you wouldn't have put up with it for an instant. It's time you stopped putting up with attacks on your body and your self-worth, whether they're coming from people you know, from strangers, or from the media and marketing industries. Here is how you do it:

Get in touch with your *healthy anger*. There are many forms of anger, and the best known and most often used ones are rage and hostility. These are not healthy types of anger because they lead you to want to take revenge on the person or thing that has infuriated you. The unthinking behavior that comes out of this irrational feeling may cause you to say or do things that you will later regret.

Healthy anger, on the other hand, doesn't use revenge as a cure; its purpose is purely self-protective. Let's look back at Angela and see how she could have used healthy anger to deal with the situation with her aunt.

Despite Angela's sincere desire and effort to change, one negative statement from Aunt Beatrice set her back into her Fat Madness cycle. The reason was that Angela was vulnerable to this type of comment. She almost *felt* it coming. Remember how she said she thought her struggle with body image felt more normal to her than her lack of struggle? The reason was that she had never learned how to respond to the outside world's appraisal of her efforts in a healthy manner.

She let her aunt's unfeeling words get to her and immediately saw herself as unworthy, inferior, and unsure of herself. She was still coming from a position of being brainwashed, even as she was trying to cleanse her mind of old junk. This set off a flood of negative thoughts and emotions that sabotaged her whole recovery program.

Suppose Angela had been prepared to respond to her aunt's comment with a healthy dose of justified anger. The exchange might have gone something like this:

AUNT BEATRICE: Dear, you really are looking better. As soon as you lose some weight in your legs, you'll look terrific.
ANGELA: Actually, Aunt Bea, I'm pretty happy with the way I

look now. I'm eating right and exercising every day. In fact, if you want to consider trying the program I'm on, I'd be more than happy to tell you about it.

I'll guarantee you that if Angela would have responded to her aunt this way, she wouldn't have had any problems sticking to her recovery program. The reason she couldn't was because she wasn't prepared to react. She didn't know how to get angry in response to unfeeling comments about her body, and that's understandable, because no one had ever suggested that she had the power to do that *all by herself, for herself.*

Don't Let Others Make You a Victim

Angela's good, healthy response would have told her aunt that first, she shouldn't make assumptions, and second, that she cared enough to help her aunt. It would have been important to let Aunt Beatrice know that she'd jumped to conclusions about Angela's own opinion of her legs. And Angela also would have let her know very directly that it might not be a bad idea for Aunt Beatrice to learn something about her own body. Angela would be kindly offering to help her do that.

Angela was justifiably angry because Aunt Beatrice was contributing to the brainwashing that she was fighting. It didn't really make any difference whether her aunt was saying this because she was a nasty, vindictive person, or because she was a person who simply never knew when she was being unintentionally cruel. The point was that Angela should have put her aunt in her place and in doing so, effectively protect herself from harm. Would there have been a tiny element of revenge in Angela offering to help her aunt recover from her own Fat Madness? Perhaps. But the desire to help would be genuine. Angela's response would not be cruel, it would be assertive.

Learning How to Be Assertive

If you are wimpy, you never get angry. You either deny the anger, and let people continue to do whatever they want to you, or you choke back your rage-filled responses and make sure that your anger never shows. If you are aggressive, you get angry whenever you please and let everyone know how unfair they've been to you. Sometimes you're angry with reason, sometimes with no reason.

But if you are assertive, you have the ability to recognize that you are being mistreated, and you also have the ability to deal with this iniquity directly. You can speak up and defend yourself and think of ways to let the other person know that *his* behavior is inappropriate and he ought to change it.

To undo your Fat Madness brainwashing, you need to give yourself some assertiveness training. The exercises that follow will give you a head start in dealing with real-life incidents. When you are prepared—as Angela learned to be—you won't feel vulnerable and you won't be in a position to lapse back into old, familiar, self-destructive habits.

The point of these exercises is to make yourself aware of times when it is appropriate to feel angry. That won't be hard. You need to give yourself permission to feel angry whenever someone makes a comment or you see an ad or a television commercial designed to make you feel miserable about your body. It is right to feel angry about an event or a statement that threatens to sabotage your efforts to recover from Fat Madness. Of course this will seem a little unnatural at first. After all, you've been programmed to respond to these stimuli with feelings of shame, self-doubt, and envy. You are going to need to practice.

Use the diary that you began in Step 4 when you were charting your hunger and satiety. You will now start a new section, entitled ''Being Assertive.'' Under today's date write:

Today, I gave myself permission to feel angry when:

1. _____

2. _____

3. _____

4. _____

5. _____

6. _____

7. _____

8. _____

9. _____

10. _____

Fill in the blanks either right after an incident occurs or at night when you have some time to reflect back on the events of the day. Here is an example of a diary filled out by one of my patients, Eileen.

Today, I gave myself permission to feel angry when:

1. I checked out the grams of fat in my "lite" margarine.
2. I heard skinny Kathie Lee talk about needing to lose weight.
3. I saw my husband watching what I ate for breakfast.
4. I saw the latest commercial for a new foolproof weight loss plan that lets you lose thirty pounds in thirty days.
5. I looked at that damn billboard with the emaciated model on my way to work.
6. Jim made that sexist comment about his latest date.
7. Gina asked me how my diet was going.

8. My mom asked me how much weight I've lost and then I told her (why did I fall into that trap?) and she congratulated me like I'd won the Nobel prize.
9. I watched a TV show, populated only by thin, young people.
10. My skinny daughter skipped dinner to lose weight.

Eileen gave herself permission to feel angry about all of these experiences, and boy, did that feel good! She didn't act on her anger each time, which shows that she had an appropriate sense of her own effectiveness in each situation. It wouldn't do her (or Jim) any good to be angry over what he said about another woman because it's not Eileen's responsibility to change the way Jim thinks. As long as his remark about his date doesn't spark any negative feelings in Eileen about herself, she's just fine. To attack his sexism would probably only get him angry and get her into a conflict she doesn't need.

But it does Eileen lots of good to get angry in situations where her Fat Madness would have formerly made her feel bad about herself. So the only items on her list worth responding to were incidents 3, 7, 8, and 10. Let's look at some appropriate assertive (not aggressive) responses to those situations.

3. I saw my husband watching what I ate for breakfast. Eileen's assertive response: "Honey, I would prefer it if you didn't watch what I'm eating. Debulking is tough enough without someone looking over your shoulder. Besides, the only one responsible for my weight loss is me."

7. Gina asked me how my diet was going. Eileen's assertive response: "Gina, I'm trying real hard to change the way I think about food and dieting. I'd be happy to explain if you're interested in hearing about my program, but otherwise, let's talk about something else."

8. My mom asked me how much weight I lost and I told her. She congratulated me like I won the Nobel Prize. Eileen's assertive response: "Mom, I answered your question because I was being polite, but honestly, I'm trying not to think about numbers of pounds lost. In the future, I'd rather deal with the weight issue by myself and not have you ask me about it. Can you do that for me?''

10. My skinny daughter skipped dinner to lose weight. Eileen's assertive response: "Honey, not eating is as bad for you as eating too much. It's a real health risk and it can seriously hurt you if you keep it up. C'mon, let's sit down and plan some healthy, low-fat meals. You can help me with the cooking.''

Do you see how assertiveness works? Assertive comments are not meant to hurt the other person. Their primary purpose is to protect your recovery and your self-esteem. They are meant to get the other person to consider what they've said and how it might affect you. You want the important others in your life to think twice before they make a hurtful statement to you. It's about time they took you seriously.

Assertive reactions don't come easily to everyone, so it's a good idea to practice at home before trying out your comments on the rest of humanity. Write down your assertive responses to the incidents you record in your diary. Don't just jump in with two feet and blurt out what you want to say before you're ready. The better you get at formulating assertive responses, the better you'll feel about yourself when you're ready to share them with others.

Deal with the Present Instead of the Past

You'll find, as you continue with this step and the steps that follow, that there are all sorts of golden opportunities to experience appropriate anger. There are lots of chances because Fat Madness brainwashing is so pervasive in our society, and every time you run up against an example of it, your recovery may be threatened if you can't get angry. Cultivate your righteous anger and nourish it when you can. It is the emotional fuel you are going to need to motivate your next task in undoing the results of years of brainwashing.

That task is to start thinking about your body, yourself, and the world *in the present.* You are going to look at them from a current, rational perspective, not as a trail of woe going all the way back to your childhood. This approach requires a new method of thinking—*rational thinking. Cognitive* or *rational emotive therapy* is used to treat a wide range of emotional and behavioral problems and it's particularly well suited to the needs of the Fat Madness dieter in recovery.

This type of therapy deals with the irrational beliefs foisted on you from the outside world, which cause you to fail. Your job when thinking rationally is to *transcend irrational cultural forces.* What you think and how you think are really crucial here, because your beliefs and attitudes are the source of your feelings. If you truly believe that the eighteen-year-old anorexic who is hawking diet products has a lot on the ball, you'll develop a negative attitude about your own ability to be like her. But if you can distance yourself from her pitch and take personal responsibility for your own actions, then you're in control—nobody else but you.

I'm sure you're aware that it's not what happens to you over the course of your life that makes you a coping, secure person or an anxious, unhappy one. What really determines the quality of your emotional life is the fix you have on what happens to you. If you're born in a ghetto and your father abandons you and you're in a terrible car crash that paralyzes you from the waist down, but you have the attitude that you're a survivor and you'll make it no matter what, then you're on top. If you're born in a mansion and are fed with a silver spoon and go to the best schools, but you think life is unfair and boring, you're doomed to a miserable existence.

Attitude is all. Attitude counts. Your attitude is reflected in your thoughts and beliefs. If you believe in yourself, and your attitude is basically positive, you will probably develop an interlocking system of useful, productive thoughts and beliefs. If you have a negative, self-defeating attitude and a distorted view of your body, food, and your self-worth, you have a good deal of hard work ahead of you to lift yourself out of the deeply embedded Fat Madness brainwashing you've acquired and held onto over the years.

You may find that it's easier for you to place blame, to say that this person or that event in your past is responsible for the way you feel now. There are those therapists who attempt to convince chronic dieters that their weight problem is all caused by some underlying past event that the patient has buried deep in her unconscious. Somehow, by uncovering this past event, the problem with food is supposed to get cured. This is not to say that abuse isn't a terrible thing. A person who was abused needs help to deal with the experience. But I am very concerned about the trend in theorizing that all chronic unsuccessful dieters were abused and that dealing with that abuse solves the problem. It's just not true.

Psychotherapy that digs up long-gone events may be useful for some people, but you don't need the past to change the present. Change can occur by working on your current thinking patterns and shaking them up. Actually, it's as easy as A B C.

Rational Thinking Can Help You Recover

The A stands for *antecedent event*. This is a fancy name for the incident or stimulus that triggers an uncomfortable emotion or self-defeating behavior. The B is the *belief system* that interprets the stimulus, and C is the *consequence* of that particular interpretation. Let me illustrate with an example.

A, the stimulus for my two patients, Janet and Gloria, is a television commercial for soda in which a group of young, fit, and trim people are enjoying an ecstatic, sexually charged yet innocent day at the beach.

Janet and Gloria are both single women in their twenties, both fall within the ideal body weight range, and each one hates her buttocks and thighs. Yet they respond to the same activating events with decidedly different feelings. Their B's, or beliefs that are generated from seeing the commercial, stem from their low self-esteem.

Janet responds with the belief that she is not worthy to attain the kind of camaraderie and bliss typified by these actors on television. She thinks, "I'll never be beautiful like them, so I'll never be happy like them."

Gloria responds with the belief that she has very little time left to fix herself. "Only two more months and I'll be at the beach. I *must* do something about my legs by then."

The C, the consequence of Janet's belief, is depression. Gloria's C is anxiety. Both are negative, maladaptive emotional responses that will simply perpetuate their respective Fat Madnesses.

Now it's your turn. Try out the A B C's of cognitive therapy by yourself. Let's say you are on a diet. Your husband compliments your progress, and then adds, "About ten more pounds and you'll look great."

What are some possible emotional and behavioral consequences of this stimulus?

You might feel ashamed and weak because you're sick of dieting and were thinking about quitting. But you have always believed, and still believe, that it is your obligation to please your husband, so you bite back angry words and agree with him.

Or, you might feel rage. You could yell at your husband, informing him in no uncertain terms that you don't need any more pressure than you're already feeling. You confirm your belief that all men are sexist pigs.

But the constructive method of dealing with your husband's comment is to become angry and tell him so in a way that will make him more sensitive to his own brainwashing and that will protect you at the same time. You might say, "You know, you may not be aware of how difficult it is for me to think I look great, and that's probably why you made that comment. Actually, I've made a lot of progress all on my own, and if you can't think of anything nice to say about it, then please don't say anything at all." That's a strong statement. He'll get the message.

Identify Your Destructive Beliefs to Undo Them

We all hold onto hundreds of maladaptive and damaging beliefs that are shaped and molded on us while we're being brainwashed. It would take pages to list all of the possible beliefs that you'll have to modify before you can undo your personal Fat Madness.

A typical damaging belief runs like this: ''If others criticize me about the way I look, I ought to do something about my weight.'' Is this rational? Do these people have any more access to the truth than you do—especially in the area of appearance? Certainly not.

By identifying the most destructive of your beliefs, you can get a handle on them. Then, by using rational thinking, you can turn your personal killer thoughts into allies in your war against Fat Madness. You can't believe you're wrong just because other people say they're right. You have to pay attention to your own inner signals.

When you learned to key into your body's hunger and satiety messages, you were able to control when and how much you ate. Just by paying attention to previously hidden signals, you were able to effect a change in your eating.

The same is true of your beliefs. Your belief system is always operative. It goes by itself, on automatic pilot. Most of the time, you don't notice it working because you take it for granted or ignore it.

Now it's time to listen to your beliefs. You will begin to see that certain stimuli trigger certain cognitive responses in you that create negative feelings and self-defeating behaviors about your body. If you notice the automatic thoughts that arise in response to these stimuli, you can change them. It's great to know what they are, because they can teach you a lot about your underlying beliefs.

When does your Fat Madness come directly to the surface? Think about some of the stimuli in your daily life that make you nuts about food or your body. Any time you find yourself dealing with grocery shopping, restaurants, cleaning up after your children's snacks, dieting, getting weighed, going to a party, buying clothes, or participating in other events that bring up those old, negative attitudes, pay attention to what you are thinking. Go back to your diary and write down any self-defeating thoughts that pass through your mind. These will serve as the basis for an analysis of your irrational and maladaptive beliefs.

Look at a sample page from one of my patient's diaries.

S=Stimulus   T=Thought

S: Choosing foods for breakfast
T: "I've got to get started on my diet today."

S: Trying on a pair of "skinny" shorts to see how my diet is going
T: "If I can't button these shorts, I'll kill myself."

S: Trying not to envy thin women at mall
T: "I'll never look like them."

S: Received invitation to a wedding
T: "I just can't face all of that food—and those people staring at me."

S: Grabbed Reese's miniature, ate it without thinking
T: "Now I blew it. I might as well forget the whole thing."

S: Ate lunch with Joanne who's skinny and eats everything!
T: "It's not fair that she can eat like that and I can't."

S: Husband has a roving eye at the beach
T: "He has got to stop torturing me like this."

You see, your brain goes into negative-thinking automatic pilot around Fat Madness issues. You have already done a lot of work on your negative thinking throughout this recovery program, and I'm sure your immediate reactions to situations are considerably different than they were before you started this book.

Remember how little it took to flip Angela back into her downward spiral? With just one comment from Aunt Beatrice so much good work went out the window. Angela stopped exercising and started eating junk food just because of her aunt's opinion of her legs. She wasn't able to keep up with her program because she still had a great many negative thoughts and beliefs she needed to work on. The struggle over body issues felt more normal to her—even after all her time in recovery—than the calm that came when she understood how she could control her feelings.

Working Toward Ultimate Success in Your Recovery Plan

You may be filled with hope about how well you've done with your recovery so far. I hope you are. But do you sincerely believe right now that you are capable of carrying this on for the rest of your life? Are you completely free of the panic, the fear, the humiliation, and the shame you've felt for so long? You probably still have a few dark moments of self-doubt. After all, a few weeks or months of change will not totally undo years of brainwashing. It's time to begin to understand the types of irrational and maladaptive thoughts and beliefs you need to fix. The following is a list of eight types of distorted thinking and rational thinking solutions you could use to counteract them.

1. Filtering

This occurs when you take all the negative details of a situation and magnify them while filtering out the positive details.

Example. You are at a party and you focus on the three women who look gorgeous and don't pay attention to the ten other women who are just ordinary-looking citizens.

Rational modified thinking. To reverse your tendency of filtering in your thinking, always seek balance in assessing a situation to include all of the facts, both positive and negative. That cocktail party had a lot of average bodies standing around you as well as the three knockouts. Look at them carefully. This type of modification in your perception will also serve you well in the mall and at the beach. It's interesting to think about how marketers play on this irrational tendency in our thinking by doing the filtering for us. They remove all of the average-looking people from the party before they shoot the commercial, leaving only the knockouts behind for us to envy.

2. Polarized Thinking

You see things only as black or white, good or bad. There is no middle ground.

Example. You want to lose thirty pounds. You lose twenty-two and just can't get any more off. You feel like a total failure.

Rational modified thinking. A similar balancing act will serve you well here. Think about the fact that you have lost twenty-two pounds, which is a lot of pounds. It's a real success. Think about it this way: "Yes, it would be nice to reach my weight loss goal, but if I can't, I can still say I've succeeded at doing my best." Balance. It works every time.

3. Mind Reading

You assume you know what people are thinking, especially what they are thinking about you.

Example. You get a look at a cocktail party and are sure that it's a criticism of your figure.

Rational modified thinking. The key to fixing this type of thinking is to *never assume*. We think we know what others are thinking because of our natural tendency to assume that other people think the same way we do. They don't. Find out what they're really thinking. Maybe the look was an envious glance at your dress or an expression of being nervous about getting introduced to you.

When you want to know what the significant others in your life are thinking about you, it's best to ask directly. If the people aren't that important to you, then be rational. Why assume the worst? And if they are thinking the worst, why care? Instead of feeling hurt, get appropriately angry at a world that has shaped people's thinking so that some are unintentionally hurtful to others.

4. Catastrophizing

You always read the worst into any situation.

Example. You injure your ankle and can't exercise for a couple of weeks. You predict that you are doomed to gain back all the weight you lost.

Rational modified thinking. In order to modify your thinking about this, you have to consider how often the worst-case scenario ever comes true. If you sustain an injury, that's unfortunate, but injuries heal. And they heal faster if you don't just sit around but work actively at getting healthy.

Your new rational thinking might go something like this: "Okay, I'm going to be thrown off my regular program for a couple of weeks. Maybe I could swim or lift free weights from a seated position instead of running and biking. I can minimize the damage by eating extra healthy foods until I can exercise again. Besides, this is a lifetime program. Two or three weeks of inactivity is very little time when you think about the scope of all those years I have ahead of me."

5. Control Fallacies

You feel either totally controlled by others, a victim of fate, or feel that you are completely responsible for the happiness of those around you.

Example. Your husband seems upset about his upcoming office party. You secretly feel responsible because you are fifteen pounds heavier than you were last year, and you think you'll embarrass him.

Rational modified thinking. Feeling responsible for other people's feelings and happiness is a real trap. You want to not only modify this damaging belief in yourself but also to help others close to you who may act on this fallacy.

Again, never assume. Check out your thoughts by asking. The most important factor here is checking your own tendencies to take responsibility for everyone else's happiness. You have no more control over that than they have over your happiness. Each person's feelings of contentment and satisfaction in life come ultimately from the inside.

6. Fairness

You continually focus on how things should be fair and just.

Example. You and your friend start a diet at the same time. She loses ten pounds in the time it takes you to lose four pounds. You're furious with her, with yourself, and with life in general because you think it's so unfair.

Rational modified thinking. Sure, it would be nice if the world were totally fair. Life experience teaches us otherwise. But the wish for fairness still infects our thinking and causes feelings of jealousy or rage in situations where we need to substitute acceptance and wisdom.

When your friend loses ten pounds and you only lose four, when nature gives you thick ankles and her thin ones, it won't do you any good to rage at the heavens. It will only detour you on the road to controlling what you can control, which is making the best of what you've got. Remember the old adage, "When life gives you lemons, make lemonade." Simplistic, but excellent advice.

7. Shoulding

This is when the word *should* forms too big a part of your internal vocabulary.

Example. You've been brainwashed to should yourself constantly about your body and food. You go to your best friend's dinner party and think, "I should skip the hors d'oeuvres and ask for more vegetables if I get hungry after the main course. And of course I should say I'm too stuffed to eat dessert."

Rational modified thinking. Removing the shoulds from your internal dialogue is a primary goal. Should implies that all the controls in your life come from outside. When you can switch your control system inside yourself, you don't have any shoulds. You determine the rules and regulations for yourself.

"You should skip the dessert; you shouldn't eat the hors d'oeuvres." Just exactly who handed down these shoulds? Usually parents, family, and society. Of course, some shoulds—usually those that deal with safety or not hurting others—make total sense. We'd all agree with the statement, "You shouldn't drive when intoxicated."

But here we're only concerned about shoulds that pertain to brainwashing, like, "You should eat daintily," or "You shouldn't get angry," or "You shouldn't offend others."

These shoulds offer lots of ways to keep yourself feeling insecure and controlled by others instead of learning how to take care of yourself. Watch out for the shoulds.

8. External Reward

You believe that hard work and personal sacrifice will always be recognized and rewarded by others.

Example. This one is simple. You work hard and lose weight. You can't believe the world doesn't immediately come to a stop to reward and praise you.

Rational modified thinking. It would be nice if everyone cared as much about you as you care about yourself. However, as we've noted before, life is unfair and people are primarily invested in themselves. They don't spend their time thinking and worrying about *your* sacrifices or successes. Once in a while, you'll get praise or other external rewards for your hard work.

That feels great, and you can enjoy it when it occurs. Just don't count on it.

The primary focus in your recovery is to feel good for yourself, not to look good for others.

Putting It All Together

By learning how to monitor your beliefs and by reversing your negative automatic thinking, you can begin to do your own cognitive therapy. You now have the tools to undo years of Fat Madness brainwashing.

First, remember that you need to use some appropriate anger in assertive ways to change the way you think and react to others. Feelings of doubt, insecurity, envy, depression, or guilt will throw you off track, so keep that edge. Stay a little mad.

Next, you need to track your automatic thoughts whenever they're triggered by Fat Madness–provoking stimuli. Then you need to evaluate your thoughts to see which type of distorted thinking style and beliefs they represent.

Finally, you can modify those beliefs to make your thinking more positive and productive. You'll find that as your attitudes change, your capacity for personal growth magnifies.

Understand that your beliefs don't change because you wake up one day and decide to think only good, happy, positive thoughts. In fact, you can only effect true change in yourself through a process of learning to think realistically and rationally.

The distorted thoughts and beliefs that have hung around you through the years can become history if you take every opportunity to work on them. You can undo the damage of Fat Madness. In its place will blossom real growth and a constant and loving attitude toward yourself that will not only help you succeed in your lifetime weight-control program but in every other facet of your life as well. After all, that's what recovery is ultimately about: learning how to live better than you ever have.

Ten Positive Affirmations to Live By

1. Everybody doesn't have to love me.
2. It's okay to make mistakes.
3. I don't have to control everything.
4. Only I am totally responsible for me.
5. I can handle it when things go wrong.
6. It's best to try.
7. I am always capable of doing my best.
8. I can change when I need to.
9. Other people can handle meeting their needs.
10. I can be flexible.

◼ STEP 8: REPAIR

I Will Take Care of Myself for Myself

How does the word *selfish* strike you? Immediately, you think of Scrooge, or of a nasty little spoiled brat hurling a toy across a room. You think of Aunt Beatrice making comments about your legs so she'll feel better about her own weight problem. You think of numerous other relatives and friends and colleagues at work. You never think of yourself.

That's the point. Most chronic dieters aren't selfish. Unlike addicts, who tend to live in a cocoon of their own needs and pleasures, the dieter always puts everyone else first. "I'm losing weight to rekindle my husband's interest in me; I'm losing weight so my kids won't be ashamed of me; I'm losing weight so I can look reasonably good at Maryanne's wedding."

A dieter's true feelings about herself get buried so deeply, it's usually impossible to find them. The food and the body are such overwhelming concerns, they cancel out all the other feelings. What an awful thing to do to yourself—to stop caring enough about you, to stop being good to yourself.

But just as expressing appropriate anger is a healthy gesture in your recovery, so is allowing yourself to be appropriately selfish. Selfish—not in terms of rejecting others, but in terms of repairing the damage you've done to yourself over the years.

This isn't going to be easy for some of you. Many addicts find that the most difficult negative emotion to shake in the recovery process is guilt, and this is certainly true of the chronic dieter. If you consistently deny yourself all pleasures, if you feel guilty every time you make yourself feel good, you won't just be able to turn around blithely and act appropriately selfish. But you're going to have to try, because it's a very important step in your recovery process.

Making Amends to the One You've Harmed—Yourself

An addict typically hurts other individuals. He's so bound up with getting what he wants when he wants it that he lies, steals, cheats, and takes advantage of those he loves. In the course of his recovery, he comes to understand that part of his work is to make amends to those he had harmed.

The recovery from Fat Madness requires making amends as well, but not to other people. Being a chronic dieter with body-weight preoccupation and low self-esteem wouldn't cause you to hurt other people, but it sure caused you to harm yourself. The time has come to make amends to yourself—because you have done yourself a gross injustice and need to make some major repairs in your relationship with yourself.

You've spent a great deal of time undoing the damage that Fat Madness brainwashing has done to your feelings and attitudes about yourself in relation to the world. Now it's time to move forward another step.

The damage you've done to yourself falls into five categories:

1. Poor or distorted body image
2. Inability to appreciate your body as a source of pleasure
3. Feeling unattractive
4. Inability to enjoy food
5. Blaming unrelated shortcomings on your weight

You may think you are affected by only a couple of these, or that some seem to hurt you more than others, but you need to consider all of them at some point in your recovery work.

POOR OR DISTORTED BODY IMAGE

There have been many studies done that show unequivocally that most dieters have no conception of their own size and shape. Though numerous experiments it has been proven that these people grossly overestimate how large they are. This distorted image simply compounds the problem of feeling fat. Not only do dieters typically abuse themselves by living under the domination of the numbers on that cruel scale, they further lower their self-esteem by truly believing that their body or certain body parts won't fit through most front doors. This false perception can be repaired. It just takes a little work.

Your exercise to establish a realistic perspective on your body has to do with shifting your focus from looking good to feeling good. Now that you have a new goal of long-term, lifetime weight control and have abandoned your old, unrealistic goal of magically turning yourself into a Madison Avenue anorexic teen model, you are ready to start working on feeling good about the way your body *actually* looks, not the way you used to think it *should* look. If you don't remember how to do this, go back to the last step and practice getting rid of some more of your shoulds.

You can only feel good about the way your body looks when you use your personal assessment that you control as your barometer, not what Uncle Harry thinks, not what the President thinks, not what the billboard on the highway tells you you're supposed to think. If you try to gauge what looking good means by using someone else's criteria, you automatically lose. There are no objective, external criteria that count.

If you look at the ideal of female beauty in various different countries, you see a huge culture gap. Typically, in underdeveloped nations, obesity is associated with the upper classes and thinness is associated—of course—with the poverty-stricken. In India or Nigeria, for example, or among the Australian Aborigines, you would be hard-pressed to win the Most Gorgeous Award if you were built like Cindy Crawford. Amazingly enough, non-Western women tend to abandon their own cultural ideals after they've moved to the United States and have been subjected to the same systematic brainwashing about thinness.*

Speaking of brainwashing, you may remember that even Cindy Crawford sees herself as big as a moose next to the anorexic models she works with.

Photo Essay: Toward a Better Body Image

What exactly is your view of your body? Can you objectively see yourself as others see you? Of course not. Your view of your body is already distorted by the unfortunate fact that your head is firmly attached to your body, so one source of distortion is the inability to see your body from all sides and angles.

Exercise 1: Home photos. You can see yourself better by looking at photographs. Have someone you like and trust take some pictures of you from the front, the back, and the sides. Wear something you feel good in. Examine these photographs as though they were pictures of someone else. Take your ego out of it, if you can, and don't let Fat Madness rear its ugly head. Try to be detached and objective. Do you really look as fat as you think? I know the answer can be difficult. Many people with Fat Madness avoid taking a hard look at themselves. But if you have courage, you can do it. It takes courage to change.

Believe me, if you walked into some model's house first thing in the morning and starting taking home snapshots with a regular old camera, the model would look no better, no worse, than any ordinary girl in the street—probably just much taller

*Mandy McCarthy, Ph.D., "The Thin Ideal, Depression and Eating Disorders in Women," *Behavior Research Therapy,* Vol. 28, No. 3, 1990.

and skinner. But the models never get the snapshot camera treatment. The type of photo you see in magazines is done in a studio with special lighting (which accentuates certain angles of the body and downplays others), costume, and makeup. It also involves a highly skilled photographer who is paid big bucks to make people look not as they actually appear, but as the advertiser wants them to appear. In these pictures, painfully thin young girls are instructed to pose with legs crossed and hips turned to create the illusion of one perfect, lean line from head to toes.

Exercise 2: Fashion shot. If you want to see what illusion can look like so that you can compare it with reality, get yourself a fashion photo. One of the most popular stores at my local mall takes glamorous pictures of very ordinary people. The results are astounding. With the right makeup, hair, lighting, and camera angles, these photographers make you look like you just stepped off the pages of *Vogue*. The experience of posing may give you a greater understanding of what this image-making business is really all about. It probably will boost your ego considerably when you see that you, too, can look like a fashion model under the right conditions.

Exercise 3: Comparison photos. Your next step in repairing your body-image distortion is to take your pictures and compare them to pictures of other ordinary people. To get really objective, you can use a ruler to measure parts of your body and compare them to other people in similarly sized pictures. Have you been too hard on yourself? Is your image of your body distorted by years of Fat Madness? Most people find the answer to be a resounding yes.

Now you can admit to yourself that you haven't been a good objective judge of your body. The exercise with the pictures can help correct that distortion, although of course, it won't totally fix it. Body image is more than just visual. It relates to your whole attitude about yourself, so now we'll work directly on correcting distortions in the way you think and feel about your body.

Thinking About Your Body

What exactly *is* your body? Most people who suffer from Fat Madness think of their body as a burden or hindrance to happiness. They lose sight of the fact that the body is also an absolute wonder of nature.

We tend to take the incredibly complex workings of the human body for granted until something goes wrong—until we become sick or injured or until our feelings about our body are changed by some external force. My friend, Jim, describes it this way.

"I hated how I looked for most of my life, and I blamed all my problems on my body. I was really hung up on it. I've been on and off diet and exercise programs it seems like forever, but they never worked. I even remember praying to God that I would wake up one morning and be magically transformed into a hunk of muscle. That was all before the auto accident where I was hurt very badly and wasn't expected to walk again.

"Throughout my entire rehabilitation, I didn't give a single thought to the desire to be thin and muscular. Not once! All I thought about and prayed for was to be able to walk again. Thank God that wish came true. Funny thing now is that I view my weight and body problem from a very different perspective. It just doesn't seem all that important anymore. I still want to be thinner and healthier, but I'm not the least bit hung up on how I look. I'm too busy being grateful that I can walk. I guess I got to learn the hard way how to prioritize."

It doesn't require a serious illness or accident for you to repair your own body image. All it takes is a new slant on your thinking. Start with what you take for granted.

Exercise: Admiring the human machine. Spend one day concentrating on your body's incredible complexity and beauty as it coordinates all your functions and processes. Walking, talking, feeling, enjoying, laughing, digesting, understanding—these are all made possible by your personal biological machine. No matter its shape, size, or color, the fundamental machinery is workable and wonderful for every one of us.

Stop and look at the articulation of your fingers, grasping and releasing. See how your balance works when you climb a flight of stairs. Stand on one foot and then another. Open your mouth and say a few words. Find out exactly what your equipment can do. I think you'll have a greater admiration for and appreciation of this extraordinary house you've been designated to live in. Clearly, you haven't been paying enough attention to your own God-given gift—yourself.

We don't think about our body as a gift because we have it hanging around all the time and we're used to it. Familiarity has bred a lot of contempt, particularly if we're always picking ourselves apart. But when you look at this miracle of form and function clearly and rationally, you can see that its weight and shape really can't make as much difference as you may have believed it did. I am asking you to stop taking your fabulous body for granted *for one day*. Spend the day thinking like a child who is driven by curiosity and delight to explore every nook and cranny and who ends up being floored by the wonder of it all. Then answer the following two questions:

1. I learned today that some of the things I take for granted about my body are: _____

_____

_____

_____

_____

_____

2. This has changed my thinking about how my body looks in the following ways: _____

_____

_____

_____

_____

You can repair the damage. And once you can think about this body that has been bestowed on you, you can really start to enjoy it for what it is instead of hating it for what it isn't.

INABILITY TO SEE YOUR BODY AS A SOURCE OF PLEASURE

Do you remember the last time you came home from work and you felt like being nice to yourself for no reason? You just relished the idea of taking a hot bubble bath and pouring yourself a glass of wine and then bundling up in a soft bathrobe and curling up with a book and your favorite music playing in the background. There wasn't anyone you needed to share this with. It was a purely hedonistic, comfortable—dare we say the word?—selfish time that was all yours.

I would be willing to bet that you don't plan these evenings for one very often. People who are victims of Fat Madness simply don't feel it's right to be nice to themselves. They are convinced that they don't deserve this kind of royal treatment.

Our body image so often interferes with our willingness to take advantage of and indulge in the many pleasurable activities that require a healthy unself-consciousness. We can't be embarrassed about our bodies if we really want to cherish and nurture them. This is exceptionally hard if you cover up not only feelings but body parts so that no one (yourself most of all) can see them. Sandra describes it this way:

"I can't tell you how many times I've wanted to sit in the communal jacuzzi at my health club after a hard workout. But I just can't be seen in my bathing suit in public, so I skip it. It's funny. I've overcome my embarrassment about being seen in workout clothes. I think that's because I still feel covered up. But letting it all hang out in a bathing suit? No way. It's such a shame though, because everyone tells me the jacuzzi feels great. Of course, they also enjoy a nice hot shower at the club, and I haven't been able to conquer that one either because I'd have to take off my clothes and put on a towel and walk to the shower stall like that. I couldn't manage it. So I still drive home all sweaty to take my shower in private."

Sandra, and so many others like her in the grips of Fat Madness, miss out on these simple but highly enjoyable little pleasures of life. The brainwashing she's endured for years has taught her that she should be so ashamed of her less-than-perfect body that she cannot show it in public. (Of course, the American Puritan ethic has accomplished a lot of brainwashing on its own by letting us know that naked is naughty and always has something to do with sex, so we should avoid it unless we're really willing to take the consequences. This damage, too, can be repaired. At this point in your program, you have learned enough and feel sufficiently better about yourself to do it.

In order for you to understand just how to be nice to yourself, you have to grasp some elemental concepts of biology. The human, as you're probably aware, is a very advanced animal. All animals exhibit certain instinctual behaviors designed to ensure the survival of the species. Among them are eating, sleeping, procreating, and for many species, caring for the young.

What motivates animals to do these things? What convinces them to eat, sleep, fight off enemies, and reproduce themselves? Within the brain matter of all animal species, there exists a special group of cells that give a feeling of pleasure to the animal when he performs certain behaviors. This special group of cells is, in fact, called *the pleasure center*.

You've got a pleasure center, too. We all do. It makes you feel good when you perform certain species survival behaviors such as eating and procreating. But it's a lot more refined for humans because we're a lot more sophisticated than other animals. We have learned to utilize our pleasure center to reward many other behaviors. The pleasure center is such a powerful motivator that some people devote their lives to stimulating it artificially with chemicals. We call these people drug addicts.

However, the pleasure center does a lot of good for most of us who know how to regulate it. We get rewards from the center for a whole host of activities like reading a good book, hearing a good joke, or watching our kids graduate from high school. Simple pleasures (some of which you may have forgotten) also stimulate this center. What about having a massage, sunbathing, taking jacuzzis at a health club, or reveling in the delight of someone else's body as you touch and hold one another?

If you're in the grips of Fat Madness, it may be difficult to allow yourself all the pleasures you deserve. Let's work on the following exercises.

Getting Your Fair Share of Pleasure

Why can't Sandra take a shower or a jacuzzi at her club? Why can't you? Do you feel so embarrassed about your body that it is physically impossible for you to show it to anyone else or to allow anyone else to touch it, even in the dark?

This is criminal. Think back to what you learned in Step 7 about using healthy anger. I want you to take your justified anger and let yourself feel it right now. Why shouldn't you get to enjoy these things? Because society has made you feel that there's something wrong with your perfectly wonderful body? The hell with them! Life is not a rehearsal. Stop waiting for tomorrow when just the right amount of weight loss will make you feel less ashamed of showing your body in public. Remember, by society's standard, that tomorrow will never come. There will always be imperfections that need fixing.

The Gorgeous Model Look-Alike Contest is a game with no winners. Make yourself a winner by choosing not to play.

Now, you can start your pleasure exercises.

Exercise 1: Enjoy the pleasures you've been missing. Make a list of all the things that you have denied yourself out of shame—going to the beach, taking an exercise class with other people, having a facial, having a sauna or a massage at the club, getting undressed and trying on clothes in the communal dressing room at your favorite department store. Pick the easiest one and make a date with yourself to go and do it within the next two weeks.

The idea may sound repellent to you right now, but you have two weeks to get used to the notion. You're always frightened when you attempt something new because it's unusual. Certainly an exercise like this one, which involves an activity you've forbidden yourself for so long, will seem like a gigantic hurdle until you've actually taken that deep breath and allowed yourself to try it.

If you pretend to feel brave, and act as though you have nothing to fear, sometimes the very bravado you exude can give you the courage you need to take the step. As Winston Churchill so rightly said, "The only thing we have to fear is fear itself."

Once you've taken a shower at your health club, for example, it's not so frightening. It's actually okay—maybe even nice. Once you've discovered that it's possible for you to take this first step (and that you even enjoyed it), make an appointment for a massage, or schedule a time for a jacuzzi or sauna. Put on your suit and go to the beach or pool.

The feelings of terror about showing yourself to others can be overcome in one glorious act of personal courage. You can repair this damage. Use all the tools you have learned in previous steps to reinforce your courage, then tear down the barriers society has set up that have prevented you from enjoying the one and only body you have.

Now we'll move on to the really tough pleasure issue: sex. This is obviously a more complex and involved topic than taking jacuzzis and going sunbathing. However, many of the same principles of repair apply. Fat Madness affects people's sex lives in multifaceted and devious ways, but it no longer has to.

In order to enjoy a healthy sex life, you must first feel comfortable in your body and then feel comfortable when someone else touches your body.

Fat Madness does severe damage in both areas. One of my patients, Roger, put it this way: "It stops me cold. It's not like I can't perform or don't want sex—I do! It's just that I can't imagine someone getting turned on touching my body. Even at times when I've lost weight, I still think this way. I have a soft belly and big love handles, and they don't go away, no matter how many pounds I shed. I can't believe they call those ugly hunks of flesh love handles. They certainly haven't done anything for my love life."

Every sense is affected by Fat Madness. For some people, like Regina, being seen is as difficult as being touched. "When Jim wants to make love with the lights on, we always end up having a big fight," she told me. "I can't. I never let him see me naked. I'm afraid if I do, I'll lose him. But the fights we have about keeping the lights on make me worry about losing him, too. I can't even consider it, so nothing changes between us, and even if we do end up touching, it's awkward and unpleasant. Sometimes, the whole effort is aborted before it's even begun."

Human sexuality is a very complex phenomenon. It's tough enough learning to deal with another person on this very sensitive level without carrying around all that mental baggage that society has forced on you.

How are you going to keep Fat Madness from interfering with your love life? You must learn to relax, get comfortable with your body as it is, and go with the flow. Relaxation exercises and training can really make a difference in our hectic and demanding world. It's unfortunate that you have to learn something that's supposed to come naturally, but after practicing these exercises for a while, they will seem like they've always been part of you.

Exercise 2: Positive imagery. Give yourself a place and a time to get into the mood. You should allow at least twenty minutes of privacy for this exercise. First, empty your mind of negative or troublesome thoughts or images. Think of wrapping them up in a sheet somewhere inside your brain and then open a hole at the top of your head and draw the sheet out, being careful not to spill any thoughts. Now you have a blank sheet. Next, imagine a peaceful scene or a lovely experience you can conjure up from your past to help relax your mind. Go over each detail and see what pleasure it brings you. You can use this technique to relax yourself before potentially stressful experiences.

Exercise 3: Deep breathing. Focus all of your attention on the process of breathing. Close your eyes and inhale slowly, taking the air in through your nose, allowing it to circulate up around your head and through your lungs. As you exhale, think of the breath filling all the spaces in your body with energy. Next, inhale from the soles of your feet and draw it up your spinal column. Work the breath up your body slowly, stopping at every organ and system. Think of the energy going up your back and down your front. You can count your breaths or simply try to empty your mind of all thoughts while you focus exclusively on restful, healthful breathing.

Exercise 4: Letting go of muscle tension. You are going to tense and then relax different muscle groups in your body sequentially. Start with the muscles in your toes and tighten them, then release them. Move to your ankles, your shins, your knees, your thighs, your perineum and groin, then work your way up to your waist, your lower torso, your upper torso, shoulders, arms, hands, neck, and head. Once you have isolated each body part, tighten your entire body and hold it for a count of five, then release it all. Feel the energy flood you.

Use these relaxation techniques daily, and you will really start to get comfortable with your body as you discover its different parts, potentials, and feelings. Does your right leg react more than your left? Switch sides. Do you feel sensations where you were numb before? Do you feel tingling in your limbs? Don't be afraid of it, but let it in. Concentrate on where those awakened body parts are.

You may find that these exercises bring up a lot of emotion in you. That's because you've had your body bottled up for such a long time and now you're freeing it. It's okay if you feel angry, weepy, or even slightly giddy.

Try these exercises clothed at first. Then take your clothes off and see how different you feel when you do them naked. Turn on a fan and let it blow over your skin while you do your exercises. Take a hot bath and feel the wonder of the warm water flowing around you as you breathe.

You can also do these exercises (no one will know) while you're in the jacuzzi with other people or lying on the massage table being treated to a rubdown. This is yet another level of intimacy that will give you greater comfort with your body and will prepare you for the ultimate intimate experience, sex.

Sex and Making Love Are Experiences You Deserve to Enjoy

If you can feel okay with your body while you're alone or in a public setting like a health club, you may be ready to trust another person with your body. When you approach a sexual encounter relaxed, you can let things progress naturally. You can stop anticipating what you *should* look like or *should* feel like and simply enjoy yourself. I can assure you that the quality of your sex life (or anyone else's) has little to do with what kind of body you have. What counts is how you feel in your body and how your sense of comfort with your body allows your partner to feel comfortable and sexy, too. I guarantee you that this is the true key to sexual satisfaction.

Don't be discouraged if the relaxation program does not accomplish what you want it to. Remember, you have years of ingrained hatred and loathing of your body to overcome, and these simple techniques may not be enough to undo the damage. There are many books that deal specifically with this problem, or you may wish to consider professional help. There is nothing to be concerned about and everything to be gained by talking to a therapist who understands the deeply rooted fears that can cause sexual dysfunction. In most cases, short-term therapy is enormously effective in this area.

FEELING UNATTRACTIVE

I wrestled long and hard to find a way to repair the damage of feeling unattractive, because I'm determined that you not play right into the hands of the enemy. The need to feel attractive is one of the primary tools of manipulation used by the multi-billion-dollar cosmetic and fashion industries. They use this device to foster dissatisfaction and Fat Madness. But the desire to look good has been with humankind for centuries, so we can't just write it off as pure victimization by the media.

It's vital to find a middle ground where the issue of attractiveness can be placed in a reasonable, undamaging personal perspective. To do that, we must explore the concept of attractiveness, and what it really means.

The word attractive is derived from the verb, "to attract." Magnets attract and so do people. To attract someone means to get his interest and attention. When this is applied to members of the opposite sex, it usually implies a sexual interest, so the first thing to find out is whether the desire to feel attractive is really a desire for sex. My patient, Susan, thought long and hard about this.

SUSAN: Sure, I like to try to look really hot when I go out. I love it when I walk into a room full of men and heads turn. But I don't want sex with any of those men. That's not what it's about at all.
DR. SINAIKIN: Then what is it all about?
SUSAN: (*smiling*) You know, I'm not really sure. I just know its makes me feel good—and a little powerful.

Men and women view their attractiveness differently. So we must examine the other side as well before we can come to any conclusions. I discussed this topic with Tim, another patient of mine. He told me, "I like to think of myself as a fairly liberated man. I really do respect women. But whenever a woman walks by, I can't stop from turning my head and checking her out. I really do undress her with my eyes. It makes me feel a little bit like a pig, but I do it. I don't know if it's just something I learned from cool kids when I was a teenager or whether my first inclination when I see a woman is, 'Could I have her if I wanted her?' I'm not into casual sex, but if one of those women walked up to me and asked me to go home with her, I don't think I could resist. Of course this is all theoretical—it never really happens."

The reason it doesn't happen has little to do with Tim and a lot more to do with why women really want to turn those heads. Go back and see what Susan said: power. It gives her a sense of power to know that she can make all the men in a room desire her to the exclusion of every other woman in the room. So it isn't just power for Susan, it's also competition.

Women are constantly engaged in a war with other women. It's a war where the victor is the best-looking woman in the club, the party, the church.

Tim, in his own masculine way, also has a war going on. He'd be devastated if Susan approached some other man in the room and invited *him* over to her place. Because, in fantasy, at least, Susan already has selected him. Tim turns his head because he really is interested in sex. He's checking out a body and face that he might want to have physical relations with. He doesn't necessarily have to pursue that goal, but it does occur to him in fantasy that it *could* happen if the circumstances were right, if all systems were go, if there weren't any better-looking, more muscular men in the room. Competition, once again.

Think about our society for a minute. We are raised on the notion that we have to beat the other guy. All that counts is being number one, the best. In a very real sense, anything less than first place is losing. Think about those shots of the losing team's locker room after the Super Bowl. Grown men crying real tears because they were merely second best out of twenty-eight teams, not first. And if you happen to be the placekicker who missed the forty-four yard field goal that could have won the game—well, suicide might be a consideration.

Raised on a diet of this kind of cutthroat battling for position, it's no wonder we all find ourselves fantasizing that somehow we could be the one and only Number One. How do we compete? Well, here it gets pretty sexist. Boys and men typically have many different arenas in which to fight their battles, from the gridiron to the board room. Women increasingly join them in both areas; however, sports and business aren't the first arena of competition for most women. From their earliest days, little girls hear parents, aunts, and uncles say, "How pretty she is! Look at her adorable tiny fingers! Look at that gorgeous face!" There's another, much bigger arena.

Things have clearly been changing for the better over the past ten years, but old habits die hard. The primary arena for most women's competition is the way they look as opposed to the way other women look. The competition can be dirty and downright cruel.

What a trap for the chronic dieter! What a source of agony for an already damaged sense of self-esteem! If you are really committed to your recovery from Fat Madness, you have only one choice. Don't enter the arena. Don't play the game. Let it go.

I am not suggesting that you shouldn't feel attractive or that you shouldn't do whatever makes you feel better about yourself, whether it's wearing makeup or dressing a certain way. I am only warning you against trying to look like those artificial representations of gorgeous that society deems worthy of showing in ads and movies. When you let go of your insistence that you have to compete with the likes of a supermodel, you reaffirm your choice to feel good *for you* and just for you.

Stop checking everyone else out; stop constantly comparing yourself to others. Choose your clothing or your look because you like how it looks and makes you feel. This is what my patient, Sylvia, said about it:

"I could never figure out if I looked good or not. I was always either soliciting opinions from other people or comparing myself to everyone else. I can remember times when I actually thought I looked good until I went out somewhere. Inevitably, I'd focus on one or two gorgeous, skinny women and compare myself to them. I'd never compare myself to the other, more normal-size women. Frankly, I don't even know if the ones I called pretty were actually pretty by society's standards. I just thought people automatically got pretty and looked happy if they were skinny. And as soon as I started the comparison, I'd immediately get that sinking, ashamed feeling.

"As I began the hard work in my recovery, though, this was the area I concentrated on. It was real hard to take care of myself, just for me. First thing I did was to go through my clothes and get rid of all the things that I really was never going to fit into. Then I bought some new outfits all by myself. I didn't take anyone else along to tell me how I looked.

"Mostly, regardless of what I wear or how I do my hair, I think it's the change in attitude that makes me feel better. I give myself a pat on the back before I go out the door every day. I tell myself I look good and leave it at that. I don't harass myself all day about it and I don't compare myself or compete with other women. It's one of the nicest presents I ever gave myself.''

Give yourself the same present. You'll never regret it. Take care of yourself for yourself. You're the only one who counts.

INABILITY TO ENJOY FOOD

What? Get pleasure from eating? But surely you've convinced yourself that over the years, the only pleasure you ever allowed yourself was the guilty one of consuming food, and that's not supposed to be important if you aren't suffering from Fat Madness. Right?

Wrong. You are supposed to like to eat. Eating is an experience that can be stimulating, comforting, and just plain fun. Believe me, most people who are victims of Fat Madness do not find food fun. They are obsessed by it, preoccupied by it, but it sure isn't delightful to eat if you worry all the time about how much weight you'll gain.

You have progressed far enough in your recovery to take a giant leap forward in pleasure through food. It is time to be able to eat your favorite foods without guilt. You know what life is all about? Moderation. Everything in its place. Just enough. Eat a little bit of everything. Now, how do you do that?

My clinical experience with Fat Madness treatment has taught me that being allowed to eat what you want remains an important area that needs repair, even at this stage of recovery. That's because the food issue isn't just about food. It is also about family gatherings, holidays, dining out, and socializing.

One of my pet peeves with almost all weight-loss maintenance programs is their attitude toward the challenge of dealing with ''potentially dangerous'' eating events and situations. The party line is that you have to watch yourself every moment any time you find yourself in proximity to a large amount and variety of your favorite fattening foods. But you can't go through life telling yourself, "I *shouldn't*."

No matter how successful you've been with your Fat Madness Recovery Program, you need to have a strategy all ready to deal with special events and dining out. I think the best strategy is one word: Enjoy!

Really. You deserve it. You know how to eat. You know how to use hunger and satiety as your barometers, how to use portion control, exposure, and substitution to develop a new healthy relationship with food. You're aware that certain foods you could choose will be less caloric or less fat-filled than the ones you've traditionally desired. But once in a while, just because you feel like giving yourself pleasure, go ahead. Don't monitor every bite. Just eat.

Most weight-maintenance programs suggest that you handle special events as though you had mental handcuffs and a gag on. Their recommendations on control and restraint are at best laughable, at worst, cruel and unusual. When you eat out at a restaurant, you are told to avoid all high-calorie foods. You are to ask the waiter to ask the chef to prepare your fish or chicken without butter, oils, or sauces. You are to order a side of steamed vegetables. Skip dessert. Oh, and did I mention the salad without dressing?

Their instructions should also include the following: "Concentrate hard on your envy of all of the other diners enjoying the chef's special loaded with butter and astronomical numbers of calories. Make sure that you feel like an outcast or a criminal being punished for having a weight problem."

That's just an evening out at a restaurant. The weight-loss people are particularly strict with you should you decide to attend a celebration, like a wedding or a family holiday. They are filled with bright advice like having a healthy, low-calorie snack before you leave so you won't be so hungry when you arrive. They caution you to stay away from the cheesy hors d'oeuvres and choose low-calorie crudités instead. And you're supposed to ask the already frazzled hostess if it's possible for the caterer to dig up a piece of plain, skinless chicken or fish rather than the prime rib that's being served to the other hundred and forty guests.

These suggestions are all supposed to be in the interests of assertiveness training. You're allowed to ask for special meals because your diet is your business. You shouldn't be embarrassed about telling the waiter about your substitutions because you're a food consumer and the waiter works for you! And you shouldn't allow your hostess or mother to force you to overeat. You don't have to have one slice of apple tart just to be polite! Be calm but strong in protecting yourself.

I'm all in favor of self-assertion, but these recommendations will *not* do anything for your recovery from Fat Madness. If anything, they will make you more self-conscious, more miserable about food, and more alienated from your body than ever. Nothing you could eat in a single evening will do any damage to your body or your recovery program if you keep that eating experience in the proper perspective. You don't need to binge. There is always another good meal around the corner.

Does it still sound impossible to sit down and enjoy a meal? Maybe you should start at the very beginning—just enjoy *a taste*. One of my patients, who, after debulking, was having a great deal of trouble getting back to normal feelings about consuming food, had started to meditate. She would take half an hour each morning as the sun was coming up to sit and be with herself quietly.

On one particular morning, after her meditation, she made herself a bowl of cereal. She mixed in some flakes and some granola and then added fresh blueberries on top. She went outside to her patio and poured milk on the cereal. Then she dug in.

But as she put the spoonful of food into her mouth, she did something very different. She focused her total attention on the eating experience. No worries about her plans or pressures for the day. Just the here and now of her body and the food. She was absolutely stunned by the explosion of tastes mixing together inside her: the crunchy flakes, the sweet granola, the moist blueberries, and the cool milk. She said it was as though time stopped and there was just that instant for her—nothing more, nothing less than the extraordinary, delicious sensation in her mouth.

You can discover this moment yourself if you get back in touch with what really counts about the eating experience. There is nothing mystical or bizarre about it. But when you are able to receive pleasure with your body, you will also be able to experience your mouth, your tongue, and your taste buds differently.

For right now, at this celebration which is part of life, for heaven's sake, just enjoy.

Of course, if you eat out or socialize around food too often, you will have to pick and choose when it comes to indulging your pleasure center. Then, obviously, you will need to exercise good, healthy eating habits most of the time and save the excesses for select special occasions.

BLAMING UNRELATED SHORTCOMINGS ON YOUR WEIGHT

We are coming to the end of your repair work. You have progressed really far in this step, so I think you're ready for the toughest challenge, which I've saved for last. In order to see the necessity for this type of repair, it's useful for you to understand another parallel between recovery from Fat Madness and traditional recovery from alcohol or drug dependence.

Two of the twelve steps in traditional recovery programs involved taking what's called a "fearless moral inventory." The willingness and ability to do this can make the difference between success and failure. Let me explain the concept of a "fearless moral inventory."

One of the most difficult things for any human being to do is to take a hard, honest look at him- or herself and acknowledge his or her flaws. I don't mean physical imperfections. We're all great at acknowledging that. I'm talking about spiritual and psychological flaws. Most people find these a lot more difficult and frightening to accept. That's why we develop such potent defenses, to protect ourselves from those qualities we just can't own up to.

These defenses, however, can be life-threatening to the addict or alcoholic. If you can't say that you're a liar and cheater, that you promised time and again not to abuse a substance and then you went right ahead and did it and have some incredible reason why you did it, you're not getting one bit better. True recovery can only come when the individual honestly and courageously faces his faults and then works toward overcoming them.

Let me tell you about Paul, who, at twenty-three, came to me for treatment of severe cocaine addiction. He told me that he'd never really had a problem with drugs until his roommate in graduate school pushed him to try cocaine. Finally, Paul gave in. He said he didn't like it at first, but his roommate kept making him try more and, eventually, he was hooked.

Paul claimed that the drug was making him mess up in school and it had changed his personality. Now, he was always irritable and nasty. He told me he was convinced that if he could just get away from his roommate, he could get off the stuff. But he couldn't afford to move.

My first reaction to Paul's personal history was that he blamed everything on external forces. His roommate and his finances were the culprits. He was just a victim, manipulated by events. Then, I took a more detailed history and found out two other important pieces of information. First, although Paul hadn't had a drug problem before graduate school, he had been drinking heavily since undergraduate school. The second piece of interesting information was that he was already doing badly in school before he started abusing cocaine.

Paul couldn't begin to recover before he acknowledged his flaws. He wasn't going to get well until he was able to take an honest personal inventory.

Some problems that Paul reported were genuinely caused by his cocaine addiction, but others were not. For example, his irritability and further deterioration in schoolwork were clearly direct effects of his dependence on cocaine, but his poor school performance was of his own doing, and this started long before he was using cocaine. He'd been in such denial about his alcohol abuse that he hadn't even bothered to mention it during his initial history. One final barrier to his recovery was that he placed all the blame for his cocaine addiction on his roommate and believed that moving out would solve his problem completely.

In recovery from drugs, the addict has to recover from the way he deals with himself just as much as he needs to recover from his addiction. Paul couldn't stop abusing cocaine until he gained awareness of his own personal contribution to his addiction. He had to stop burying his head in the sand. He needed to work on his tendency to deny the existence of obvious problems (his alcoholism and poor performance in school). Also, he had to stop blaming external forces for problems that are his responsibility (his roommate, his lack of money).

Paul was guilty of both *denial* and *placing blame,* and these were both ways of avoiding responsibility. Before Paul could recover fully from his alcohol and cocaine addictions, he had to first see these problems and then be willing to work on them. Abstaining from drugs was crucial in his recovery, of course, but would never have done the job if he hadn't been able to take a real moral inventory and worked to change his character weaknesses into character strengths.

Now we return to the job of recovering fully from Fat Madness. As you can probably see, it requires a similar commitment.

From the day you came to believe that your self-worth was

directly proportional to the size of your body (the bigger your body, the smaller your self-worth), you were damaged by your belief system. And since this belief system was reinforced by society's heavy-handed message, the damage got worse.

There's another kind of damage you've sustained over the years, and this one is even more subtle and powerful. When you were told your body was flawed, and you believed it, you were handed an all-purpose tool to use for all other occasions as well. You began to blame your body for other shortcomings and problems in your life that had absolutely nothing to do with your weight. So while you were frantically busy trying to fix your body, you were missing the opportunity to work on personality traits that could have improved the quality of your life.

If you had done nothing about your body, but really concentrated on being less self-pitying, or less ego-centered, you might have eventually arrived at this same stage in recovery.

In addition, if you don't work on your personal weaknesses now, they will eventually frustrate your efforts to recover and throw you back into full-blown Fat Madness once again. The only way to fully recover from an addictive illness is to work on becoming an emotionally healthy human being who functions well in all situations. The inventory of your character traits is a crucial exercise in that process.

Exercise 1: Taking an inventory. Go back to your diary and start a new section called "Weak Into Strong." I want you to use a checklist to identify negative personal attributes that you employ in daily life.

On the following page is a list of personal weaknesses along with a list of their opposites or character strengths that you can work on incorporating into your life.

Character Weakness	Related Character Strength
1. Self-pity	Willingness to change
2. Self-importance	Modesty
3. Self-condemnation	Self-valuation
4. Dishonesty	Honesty
5. Impatience	Patience
6. Hate and bigotry	Love and tolerance
7. Resentment	Forgiveness
8. False pride	Humility
9. Jealousy and envy	Understanding
10. Laziness	Activity
11. Procrastination	Promptness
12. Insincerity	Straightforwardness
13. Negative thinking	Positive thinking
14. Immorality	Personal moral code
15. Selfishness	Generosity

Does this sound a bit like what you learned in Sunday school?
It should. These are the principles of spiritual growth—the cornerstone of recovery.

How do you use this list? At first, I just want you to identify
those weak reactions you have to daily situations. Were you
impatient with your kids today? Were you jealous of your
friend's weight loss? How could you have acted strong rather
than weak? How could you look at exactly the same situation
and perceive it positively rather than negatively?

Think about all the attributes on the list and review them daily.
You might want to take a monthly calendar and fill out the
weaknesses on the left side and the strengths on the right. Each
day you can fill in the blanks by recording whether you tended
more toward the weakness (W) or strength (S) that day. Feel
free to add any pairs of related traits that don't appear on the
list but are important in your life.

Don't Be Hard on Yourself—Repair Takes Time

There is no right or wrong here; no one is judging you, so don't judge yourself. Stop being so self-critical. The kinds of mammoth changes you are making in your attitudes and beliefs will take you time. You've got time, so use it. You are now on the path of striving toward certain goals, and you can only meet these goals to the best of your ability. Some days will be easier than others, and you may go backward a bit before you leap forward. That's normal and natural.

When you are aware that you have the potential to downplay your weak side and bolster it with your strong side, you can truly grow as a person. Hopefully, this list will help you see how working on your body without working on your soul is only a halfway measure. As they say in the Twelve-Step Program, "Half-measures avail nothing."

So go for it. Have courage and face yourself honestly. You'll like the results.

STEP 9: ACCEPT (TWO)

I Fully Accept the Results of My Best Efforts

If she was wise, your mother always encouraged you to do the best you could. You should have been comforted by that statement, because it meant that your best was an individual matter, something unique to you. It wasn't *her* best or your best friend's, or your teacher's, or the President's.

Did you fully accept that statement? Did you really appreciate the fact that all things being equal, accepting reality means that we may not do the best, but we will do *our* best? Maybe our best will only be mediocre, if it comes to that, but it will be all ours.

Achieving peace of mind about your abilities will be the most challenging task you will accomplish in your Fat Madness Recovery Program. It is essential that you start to relax and stop hassling yourself over what you cannot change. You have to stop insisting that there is more to do. Maybe there is but then again, maybe there isn't.

So here is an important question: Does Fat Madness ever end? As you get to Step 9 of your program, won't you be able to see the light at the end of the tunnel? Won't you ever reach a time and place where you will never again worry about what you put in your mouth, or obsess about how much you eat, or scold yourself about missing one day of exercise?

As you get older and hopefully wiser, will this nutsiness ease off?

The Long Hard Road of Fat Madness

Let me tell you a story. I was invited to talk about Fat Madness to the members of a local garden club. I really had no idea what the composition of the audience would be, and when I arrived, I was startled to find that everyone was over seventy years old. I figured I was in for a rough time (I hate a bored audience). In addition, I was only allotted thirty minutes for what was at least a ninety-minute presentation.

The meeting included a buffet potluck lunch where each woman brought in her favorite dish to share. A tempting array of goodies had been laid out on the table, including lots of gooey desserts. As soon as I walked in the door, the comments began.

"Oh, oh, there's the diet doctor. We're in trouble now."

"I usually don't eat like this, doctor."

"We should have brought some carrot and celery sticks."

"I just lost fifteen pounds."

"Hey, these hips aren't bad for an old lady, what do you think?"

"Doctor, what's your opinion of Jenny Craig?"

I was at once disheartened and also not terribly surprised that Fat Madness was alive and well among these women. I was upset because I felt that by now, with all the maturity and experience these people must have accumulated over the years, they should be over their preoccupation with their weight. But I was not that startled by the comments because I know this problem is universal. It starts younger and younger in our society, and extends way beyond an age where the culture demands that we be juicy, fit, and competing to look the best in a swimsuit.

The women were fascinated by my presentation and allowed me the ninety minutes I needed. They seemed desperate for some relief from their obsession, and were delighted to hear what I had to say about enjoying the bounty they had laid out for lunch.

So how long will your Fat Madness last? I think it's safe to say that it *can* last from childhood to the grave, if you don't do something about it and stay on top of it.

Getting Rid of Your Fat Madness Demons

There is a way to put some closure on this issue, to demote it from the status of obsession to the level of plain old worry, just one of life's little problems. The way to do this is to truly and fully accept the results of your best efforts. Acknowledge that you have taken charge and will stay in charge, so it's all right for you to put the issue on a back burner. There will always be a little light under it, because you'll have to stir the pot every once in a while, but it doesn't have to ignite your whole life anymore.

You can reach this stage of full acceptance by two simple methods: Practice relapse prevention and strive for serenity.

How to Practice Relapse Prevention

When the alcoholic in recovery takes one drink, when the recovering cigarette addict sneaks a smoke, when the recovering gambler bets on a football game, they have relapsed. Anyone addicted to substances and behaviors that are totally destructive and *not* necessary for survival has no business going back for just one. It's simply too dangerous. If you're addicted, just one won't do. As they say in AA, "One is too many and a thousand is not enough!"

Total abstinence is the goal that every addict has to set for him- or herself in recovery. (This is why you're never fully recovered—the process is never over—but you are always recovering.) But what about food? It isn't the same, because food is necessary to survival, so we can't abstain from it.

How do you know if you've relapsed? Before I answer that, I want to let you know that there is an organization known as Overeaters Anonymous (OA). They have made an exact translation of the original Twelve-Step Program for recovery from alcoholism to the problems of the troubled eater. They feel that any processed food that has no nutrients is dangerous and should be avoided. According to OA, any consumption of white sugar, white flour, and, for some programs, alcohol, sweets of any kind, nuts, fried foods, sugared soft drinks, high-fat cheeses, and honey is a relapse. One instance of going off course means you're bouncing off the meridians in OA.

This is such wrongheaded thinking! Take a look in your pantry and refrigerator. What doesn't contain flour or sugar? Sure, you can blame the cookies, but how can you say anything bad about pasta, bagels, and a whole bunch of other foods the USDA recommends as the new staples of healthy eating (see the Food Guide Pyramid on page 138 in Step 6)?

Abstinence from the above-mentioned foods is essential in OA, and relapse is defined as indulging in any of these "substances" (yes, this is what they call those "bad" foods). Following a relapse, you're supposed to call your sponsor, get to a meeting, and go back into a program if the relapse is out of control.

I don't buy this. I don't think that concerns about the body and problems with eating and body image directly parallel the disease of the addict. On the other hand, I think that the issues of recovery are the same, and it's perfectly possible to slide away from the path toward health.

So what is a relapse on your Fat Madness program? If you stop exercising, if you stop gauging your food intake on hunger and satiety, if you return to old, unhealthy eating habits or go right back to binging when you're depressed or elated or for any other reason, you've relapsed.

I have defined relapse in Fat Madness recovery as *gaining back five pounds of fat tissue*. Not that you're five pounds up because you've been sick or injured and can't exercise, not because of menstrual bloat, or a weekend of too much salt in your diet. But five pounds of fat. Five pounds is not too late for anything, but it is a warning that you should heed very carefully.

Relapse is an opportunity to get back on track before it's too late.

If you were addicted to self-destructive behaviors before and you don't monitor your recovery, you can get right back into those behaviors because old habits die hard. We've had them with us for so long, they're comfortable and familiar, like a pair of old slippers. They feel more right to us than any new or different ways of acting. If we slip back to these habits we were addicted to, we can just as easily lose our way along our chosen path.

Getting Back on the Program

"I really wished I'd come back sooner," a former patient named Cassie told me on her return. "I felt so good after completing the program. I felt that I finally had my insanity licked. And then I lost it. I really don't know when it happened. The madness just started coming back. Of course you can see that, can't you? I've gained back all my weight, I hate my body, and I've failed on three new diets already. Please help. I want to feel just like I felt when I finished your program. And I have no idea how to do it."

Cassie had suffered a total relapse. She lost hold of her recovery program, began to eat obsessively, hated her body, skipped her exercise sessions, and turned in desperation to commercial weight-loss programs. She said it was odd—she didn't really remember the first time she turned the alarm off and didn't get up for her morning walk, but that same day, she dug into the bag of doughnuts her husband had brought in for breakfast. It was as if her mind turned off and she kept eating without thinking of the consequences. She didn't even consider the apple with peanut butter that had become her morning staple.

When the alarm rang the next morning, she turned right over. That day, she bought a quart of ice cream after work and ate the whole thing. She said it was like a huge wave crashing over her, and one wave led the way for the next. Cassie had gained back thirty pounds before trying to diet again, but it was too late. She felt hopeless—like a real failure.

What happened to Cassie can happen to anyone, but it doesn't have to go this far. A relapse can be short-circuited before those waves overcome the seawall and the ocean pours in. If you don't let the relapse run away with you, as Cassie did, you can stay in charge. You can prevent the old Fat Madness out-of-control feelings and events once you understand the concept of the "give-up" weight.

Don't Allow Yourself to Get to the Give-Up Weight

Five pounds doesn't seem like a lot to take care of. Even ten seems manageable. But Cassie put on thirty pounds, and you know how long it takes to debulk sanely when you have that much to lose. It's so disheartening to feel that you've literally eaten up your entire accomplishment.

During years of treating patients who were addicted to yo-yo dieting, I know it's common to begin to have problems again several months after a recovery program has been completed. A chronic dieter with Fat Madness may go all the way through the nine recovery steps and then proceed to fluctuate in her ability to hold onto her new way of being and believing. Maybe she'll stick to some elements of her maintenance program and lose others. She might gain a little weight back at first, then lose again. She might continue eating sensibly for a while and keep up a modified exercise program, and then, one day, just stop.

Why is this? Is it the feeling of not deserving to succeed or the envy about how everyone else sloughs off, eats, and acts like a slug? Is it not really trusting the new body/mind-set? Who knows for sure? It's probably each of these elements and a few more. But it does happen.

At some point in recovery, a very curious and destructive thing can happen. A previously committed individual just gives up. Then the weight really starts to pile back on, until it's time for the next diet.

It's the "give-up" weight that sparks this complete abandonment of the maintenance program. Here is the typical scenario.

Joe loses thirty-three pounds following a diet. He eases off on some of the maintenance rules and quickly gains back six pounds. He's not too upset by this. He still fits into his new clothes and feels a whole lot better.

Over the holiday season, the awareness switch gets turned off in his head. He doesn't think about when he's hungry. Food is just around all the time and he feels free to indulge in it, and not to the point of satiety, either. He wants all of his favorite foods and he wants as much of them as he can get. It's suddenly too much trouble to stick with his exercise program because of holiday parties and family visits. He has a good excuse. It's just for a while, he's got to show his relatives around, and they'll be gone soon.

By now, the weight gain is creating problems. He can't fit into his new pants and has to go back to wearing some of his old ones. He starts to feel miserable; he wakes in the morning feeling leaden and puffy, and he doesn't have the energy to get through a whole day. A candy bar at 3:00 P.M. every day gives him a brief lift, but it's very brief.

The scale tells the horrible truth. He has gained back sixteen pounds. He has stopped exercising altogether and is back to his old habit of chomping chips mindlessly in front of the television. Joe knows he needs to pay attention to what he's doing before he gains back all thirty-three pounds, but he can't. He simply can't face deprivation again. Joe is on the inexorable road to gaining back all of his lost weight. He has given up.

I believe that most chronic dieters have their own "give-up" weight, that magical number of pounds regained after a successful debulking program that triggers all of the negative self-talk and destructive behaviors that send most people back down that awful road to Fat Madness. My own informal survey tells me that the give-up weight for most people lies between ten and twenty pounds.

Is gaining back ten to twenty pounds considered a relapse? No. If you've slid back this far, it's more than a relapse, it's a reversion to the chronic addictive behavior you've been engaged in all your life. *Don't let it get this far*.

You've practiced positive changes in patterns of thought and behavior throughout your Fat Madness Recovery Program. A five-pound weight regain should show you that you're not thinking and acting positive anymore. You've switched over to destruction mode, and it is time to switch back.

Remember, one episode does not equal a relapse! So what if that one time you went nuts on the appetizers at the wedding or succumbed to the temptation of an entire bag of cookies? One event does not destroy anything that you've built up so far—not your weight, not your self-esteem, not your committment to life-long health. The five-pound relapse rule, on the other hand, gives you a realistic barometer. It reminds you to be alert and to be mindful of yourself. And it's not just you. No matter how strong a program of recovery anyone has going, we are all at risk of giving up at any time.

Monitoring Yourself for Relapse

I want you to reconsider your use of the scale at this point in the program, because it can be a great help in monitoring for relapse. I am generally against scales during debulking. I think people suffering from Fat Madness tend to use them compulsively when they have nothing but pounds coming off on the mind.

But after the debulking is over, it can be really rewarding to get a new appreciation of what it means to hold your weight range. Notice I said *weight range*—a fluctuation of two or three pounds up and down is nothing to get incensed over. Start to get vigilant if it's a few pounds up for a few days.

The scale is an easier monitor against relapse than how your clothes fit. (You will remember that Jim still fit into all his new things when he was five pounds heavier.) Weighing in once a week is a good way to keep tabs on your recovery program once you've reached your goal weight.

What to Do If You Relapse

You already know what to do if you're five pounds up from your goal weight, but I'll say it anyway: Debulk! Go back on your favorite debulking program and get the pounds off. Beef up your exercise regimen. This way you won't even come close to a give-up weight.

Do you think this recommendation sounds obsessive? It's not. It's the only necessary rule you need to follow on your Fat Madness Recovery Program. I have encouraged you throughout to relax about your body and the way you handle food. But you know—and I know—that you won't be relaxed if you're unable to stay on course with your maintenance program. This is reality, and you have to deal with it. You'll start to criticize yourself and get down about your prospects of ever gaining control of your body, so it's important to take that five pounds off as soon as it goes on.

If you have regained weight, you must do more than simply debulk physically. The process, of course, is mental and emotional as well. Go back and review relevant parts of your program. Don't be surprised if the issues that need the most work are back in Step 1. If you're denying that anything's wrong, yet you've stopped exercising and started eating the way you used to, then you need to concentrate on the essentials. A return of denial always precedes a relapse, so ask yourself if you remember why you're doing this. Do you know how far you've come?

If you've been less attentive to your program lately, it's important to ask yourself why. Maybe you're under lots of stress right now, and you're looking for old sources of comfort. Maybe you aren't so threatened by overeating, and have just relaxed too much because you think you have the program completely under control.

Believe me, it's never totally under your thumb. You've never finished working at it. So, if you find yourself slipping, go back and pick up some of the cognitive therapy techniques. Go on and start a new exercise activity. Go forward and work on a relationship with someone else. Give yourself new challenges each day, and your program will never get stale.

It's very common in recovery to be weak in the essentials because we think we understand the baby steps and want to jump right ahead to the more complex issues. If we don't have the groundwork, the structure will fall. Very often, the basics seem easy when we begin. Then, after we've been through the entire process, we realize we didn't get it the first time because we missed the subtleties. Maybe rushing ahead too fast is the reason we relapse.

Of course, you can avoid needing to debulk following a relapse if you are alert for the signs that a relapse is coming, and if you respond to those signs before you've regained an ounce. If you know yourself well enough to understand how you react to external and internal influences on your self-esteem and body image, you can prevent relapse.

Relapse Prevention

I think that the most powerful recommendation in the Twelve-Step Program is, "It works if you work it." This means that the work of recovery is going on all the time, every day. And the only way to make it work is to stay in the present moment and take it one day at a time.

If you are not working your program every day, then a relapse is right around the corner. There's no middle ground: You are either in recovery or you are heading for a relapse. It's that simple.

This isn't unnecessarily strict or harsh, it's simply a fact. Recovery from Fat Madness isn't the focus of your life, but it is a part of you, and you must keep it important. When you let go of all the old myths, you must accept the truths that replace them. One is that you have a chronic condition that will need lifetime control.

What makes the program work, in the long run, is that it

allows you to boil life down to its essential elements. There aren't any outs or any valid excuses. You do have to be *with* yourself at all times. Remember the cartoon of the little boy with an angel on one shoulder and a devil on the other, monitoring everything he did? The devil encourages him to misbehave, and the angel tells him that he can do what he pleases, but he won't like himself very much if he indulges in the momentary pleasure of doing wrong.

We are all like that little boy, except that there is no devil that makes us relapse. What changes our behavior and makes us slip from our chosen path is lethargy. It's falling asleep at the wheel. It's not paying attention to what we're supposed to be doing, which is working our program every day. It is possible to stay on target and get yourself back on track well before the time when another episode of debulking will be required.

"I knew things weren't working as well as they had been on the first day of beach season," said my patient Barbara. "I thought I had progressed so much further in accepting my body. But seeing the other women in their bathing suits really threw me. I started to get that creepy feeling again, started to wish I looked like them. I started to think about dieting and I knew I was in trouble. So I went back to review Step 3. I knew I had to work on letting go some more, so that I could get some of the garbage out of my head before it started to run me again."

Barbara anticipated the problem and was able to head it off long before it got serious. She prevented her relapse by waking up to the fact that she wasn't working her program.

You can do this, too, by taking your morning walk every morning, shopping with a list all the time, and receiving the abundance of the moment each time you put something in your mouth.

Trust me when I tell you that this strategy is a winning one. Follow it, and your days of emotional suffering about your body and food will be over. All that remains will be to enjoy that extraordinary feeling that is born of the hard work you've done. The offspring of your labors is called *serenity*.

Tasting Serenity

This program has generally focused on practical, common-sense ideas, both physical and psychological. We haven't dealt with some of the deeper philosophical and spiritual issues that lie at the core of all recovery programs. In part that was because a weight problem is not in and of itself spiritually damaging, so spiritual issues may not be relevant for the person troubled about eating and food. But a secondary reason that spirituality hasn't been discussed yet is that up to now, you were dealing with the preliminary nuts-and-bolts work. You weren't ready to tackle the idea of inner peace.

Now you are. The enormous benefits you can reap from working and living your program of recovery can truly change you as an individual. They can begin to define for you what really counts. The outcome of your understanding and vigilance, the final reward of your being able to accept yourself fully, is a state of mind known as serenity.

We all know what the American dream consists of, and how much trouble it's caused us in the past. The desperation of our search for the kind of wealth, fame, and looks that we see in our sports figures, movie stars, and celebrities made us greedy for what we could never attain but were told we were supposed to want. We believed that all their flashy attributes and possessions made them happy, despite their suicide attempts, broken marriages, and other tragedies too numerous to mention.

Still, we crave anything that *looks like* the image of happiness our public figures project. That's the American dream—and it's hogwash.

Have you ever wondered what people in China, Liberia, India, Spain, and every other culture dream of? What about people who lived a long time ago? What did people dream of and strive for in 1351 or in 300 B.C.? When you think about it this way, you understand that the values you've been taught to cherish are ephemeral and meaningless. What you want today wouldn't remotely interest a person who lived somewhere else in another era. The very difficult notion of happiness is a philosophical concept, and it's completely relative to the culture that educates you and drums its particular definition into you.

One aspect of the American definition of happiness has been very hurtful to you. It has made you anything but happy, and I'm sure you know that I'm referring to your idealization of a certain look. That impossible dream has gotten you into your Fat Madness, and you've worked very hard to extract yourself from it.

I'm sure that people in every culture and in every time can point to equally hurtful aspects of their particular cultural definitions of what constitutes happiness. We recognize that happiness isn't precisely what the culture says it is, so we can redefine what we want—this time, by our *own* standards, not the culture's.

A lot of people have spent a lot of time trying to come up with a definition of happiness that transcends time and space. Many great thinkers have arrived at the conclusion that we can never achieve any lasting happiness, and searching for it is just a trap. The great religions of both East and West agree that a more realistic goal in human life is to strive for contentment, wisdom, and charity.

In Twelve-Step Recovery Programs, which incidentally thrive in remarkably diverse cultures, this wisdom is expressed in the Serenity Prayer:

> *Grant me the serenity*
> *To accept the things I cannot change*
> *The courage to change the things I can*
> *And the wisdom to know the difference*

This timeless piece of advice shows you exactly what the Fat Madness Recovery Program can do for you when you believe in it and work it every day. It reminds you to accept yourself fully—and this includes all the aspects of yourself you can't do anything to change. You must accept that you have done the best you can to make your body healthy and attractive to yourself, that you live in a culture that worships thinness, and that life isn't always fair.

The prayer tells you to have the courage to take control where you can by having the courage to rise above the petty concerns of your culture, define your own code of self-worth, and learn to like yourself—maybe even love yourself.

Finally, you must pray for the wisdom to make a distinction between the things you must accept and the things you can have control over. The pursuit of this wisdom will last you a lifetime. It never ends.

In the Eastern philosophies, we are told that we are all traveling along a path or "the way." Do you ever get there, or are you always on that path? A journey of a thousand miles, says the Chinese philosopher Lao-tzu, must begin with a single step. You have taken that first step—and at least eight more.

The Benefits of Meditation

You can call it what you will—prayer, meditation, silent communion with yourself—but it's a real boost on your path to serenity. If *prayer* seems too religious a concept to go along with feelings you have about your body, then maybe you want to call it *deep thought* or *getting in touch with your inner space*. Whatever you call it, it works.

Meditation—another name for this experience—helps to empty the mind of clutter and allows you to focus on what's important. When you have meditation as a part of your life, you can be serene in the face of chaos, hurtful comments, and cultural stereotypes. Allowing the mind to settle is a technique that has worked for mankind for thousands of years in hundreds of cultures, and it may work for you as well, even if you've never prayed or meditated before. There's really nothing simpler, and you don't have to be a deeply spiritual person to be able to focus on one thought, one sound, one breath—and ultimately calm yourself inside and out.

Give yourself fifteen minutes at first, and work your way up to half an hour. You need a quiet, well-ventilated place with no distractions. Sit cross-legged on the floor, or in a straight-backed chair if you need support. Close your eyes and get comfortable, but not so comfortable that you feel like you're falling asleep. The meditative state aims for heightened awareness and a vital, active feeling throughout your body and mind.

Begin by taking deep breaths, feeling that each time you exhale, you are sending out bad or confused thoughts, and each time you inhale, you are taking in warm, healing waves of energy. Keep your breathing even, taking air in through your nose and letting it out through your nose and mouth. Think about sending the breath to all parts of the body.

Some people like to meditate on one sound, such as "om." Some like to imagine an exchange of energy from the outside to the inside. And some like to clear the mind completely of all thought. This is rather advanced stuff, so don't feel embarrassed if, when you first start meditating, you find you have a hundred thoughts racing through your mind. Let them pass, say good-bye to them, and then comfortably settle into yourself. Eventually, you may experience something you've never known before— peace of mind.

Sharing with Others: Giving Charity

The final concept in your recovery is charity. When you are confident about the way you handle food, and when you begin to feel better about your body just as it is, you are going to face two spiritual challenges. The first is the one we have discussed throughout this book: You must be strong in the face of the forces constantly at work trying to knock you off your path to recovery.

The second challenge will be to reach outside yourself to others. As you well know, you aren't the only person around with obsessive concerns about the body and food. In order for you to work your recovery each day, you have to extend yourself beyond the bounds of your own body and mind to reach other people.

Fat Madness is all around you. You don't have to look very hard, because it comes right up and smacks you in the face when you're attuned to it. As Barbara noted, "I never realized how miserable everyone is with his or her body. I guess that was because I was right there with them. But I see it now, and I can't believe it. There isn't a single meal or after-work conversation where fat and dieting isn't the main topic. People are preoccupied with their physical bodies, and no one is happy with what they've got, whether they look fat or thin or attractive or whatever.

"It's more than being dissatisfied, though. I think everyone is in turmoil. No one can accept what they're really like. I feel sorry for people who hate themselves so much and try every means to get what they can never have. I want to help them, but I really don't know how."

My advice to Barbara and to you is to stay humble. Don't get preachy and proselytizing. Don't become the kind of person who has hurt you for so long, someone who feels superior to fat people. Even though you may feel right now that that you'd never become smug about your success and your recovery, be on guard.

Charity means that you offer assistance and care to others just like you. In so doing, you will help yourself by helping those around you who are still suffering. Remember how you always hated those obnoxious idiots who'd just lost twenty pounds on some brilliant plan or other and had to shove it down your throat? Don't be like that about your recovery from Fat Madness.

How do you help others, especially those whose suffering is obvious? Don't tell them; *show* them. Live your recovery and others will want to follow your example. And when they come to you and ask for your help, then give it freely and with enthusiasm. You'll never feel better about yourself.

You'll see that your body isn't the end of it all. It's not life's main show. But the serenity you achieve, the peace of mind, the confidence that you can handle any stress and rise above it is what you're here for. You're on a path. You're not aiming for one specific place, but the challenge of that path is that it can—and will—lead you to a better understanding of yourself and others.

The wonder of living in the present moment, fully accepting yourself, is that you really do have time to smell the roses. Colors will look brighter, the world and everything and everyone in it will seem more alive to you.

As you stop experiencing your body as the center of all pain and discomfort, as you work more on your mind and emotions and spirit, you'll discover to your amazement that this path leads you back to your body. You'll arrive there with no expectations or false hopes. Rather, you will be filled with wonder at all this stuff going on inside you that has absolutely nothing to do with the way you look.

When you have truly tasted the delicious fruits of serenity, you will feel the roots of your Fat Madness weakening at last. The stunted beliefs you've clung to in the past will be replaced by a lovely awareness that you're here for a reason, whatever it may be, and you can laugh and cry about it. You can really enjoy it.

It's life. And it's all yours.

Where to Go for Help

You may find, as you proceed along the path of this recovery program, that you are increasingly interested in subjects that up to now have caused you pain and misery. You suddenly see the benefit of being knowledgeable about diet and exercise because they are an integral part of your life. Here are some of the organizations that will provide you with background information and many resources:

American College of Sports Medicine
Public Information Department
P.O. Box 1440
Indianapolis, IN 46206-1440

A dollar and an SASE will get you an excellent brochure on diet and exercise regimens.

American Dietetic Association
Anderson Secretarial
1132 S. Jefferson St.
Chicago, IL 60607

They offer a variety of low-cost brochures on good eating.

Center for Science in the Public Interest
1501 16th St. NW
Washington, DC 20036

This consumer advocacy group has many excellent posters and charts on food ingredients and additives.

Americans for Safe Food
1501 16th St. NW
Washington, DC 20036

This is an adjunct organization to the Center for Science in the Public Interest.

USDA (The United States Department of Agriculture)
Superintendent of Documents
US Government Printing Office
Washington, DC 20402

The Food Guide Pyramid chart on page 138 comes from this office and there are many other excellent publications you can order on diet and nutrition.

The National Heart, Lung and Blood Institute
Superintendent of Documents
US Government Printing Office
Washington, DC 20402

This branch of the National Institutes of Health offers free publications on diet, cholesterol, and cancer through the Government Printing Office.

The Food and Drug Administration (FDA)
FDA
HFE-88, 5600 Fishers Lane
Rockville, MD 20857

They offer free copies of articles on men's and women's nutrition that have previously appeared in their journal.

The American Cancer Society
(branches in most cities)

This nonprofit organization sponsors research, education, and patient information and will send you free pamphlets on diet and nutrition.

The American Institute for Cancer Research
Washington, DC 20069

This nonprofit organization sponsors research and education programs and will send you booklets and brochures if you send them an SASE.

National Diary Council
Rosemont, IL 60018-4233

This organization is now promoting low-fat dairy selections. Ask for a booklet entitled "Wise Food Choices."